RETHINKING MEDICINE

RETHINKING MEDICINE

Harmonizing Science and Herbal Tradition

BENTON BRAMWELL ND
W MATTHEW WARNOCK JD MBA

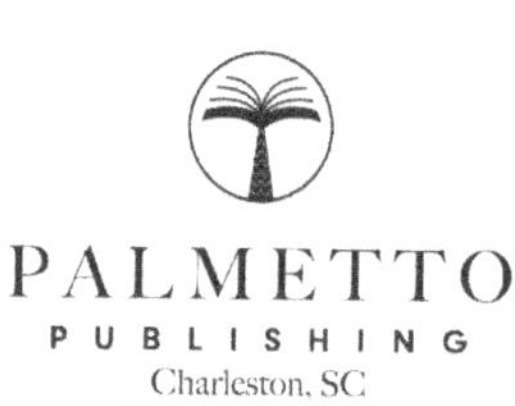

Paperback ISBN: 9798822953079
eBook ISBN: 9798822953086

Contents

Preface

This book really began in 2000 when my mother got sick. Mom was one of nearly 200,000 victims of fen-phen (a combination of two FDA-approved drugs, fenfluramine and phentermine), commonly prescribed in the 1990s for weight loss. Mom, like roughly one-third of the people who took fen-phen, developed heart problems and was given less than two years to live by her doctors. She survived until 2014, passing away within three weeks of my dad. Unfortunately, she was bedridden for most of that time due to two strokes. Despite her condition, she maintained her love for life and sense of humor until the very end, although after her second stroke, she often slept for over fourteen hours a day.

In the early 1990s, my father and a partner acquired a small line of professional herbal medicines sold directly to natural health professionals. Seeing the limited scope of this market, they chose to broaden their reach by offering these herbal remedies as over-the-counter products in health food stores. Dad's partner, Clyde StClair, had previously worked at Nature's Way, managed several health food stores, and had extensive knowledge of the natural products market. On the other hand, my dad had an MBA, an accounting background, and expertise in business turnarounds but no prior experience in herbal medicine. However, this unique pairing of skills proved successful. Together, they rebranded the formulas and established what would later become RidgeCrest Herbals. Within a few years, their products emerged as industry leaders in several categories.

In 1998 I moved from Silicon Valley, where I had spent most of my childhood, to Utah to be closer to my aging parents, among other reasons. When my mother suffered her first stroke, I stepped in at RidgeCrest so my dad could devote more time to her. Around the same time, my father's business partner, Clyde, was diagnosed with Parkinson's disease. Despite my lack of experience in the herbal industry, which paralleled my father's own beginnings, armed with an MBA and legal experience, I assumed full responsibility at RidgeCrest. My parents and Clyde faced significant health challenges, and their financial stability for retirement hinged solely on RidgeCrest's income. I felt a strong sense of duty to ensure their well-being and comfort. It was only later, after assuming this added responsibility, that we bought out Clyde.

In the beginning, with an attorney's mind, I faced one overwhelming concern: if a combination of two FDA-approved drugs could cause problems like those associated with fen-phen, how could I be sure our products wouldn't do the same? After all, our products weren't FDA tested and our formulas combined dozens of herbal ingredients. How could I be sure they were safe? I envisioned litigators lining up at courthouses across the country, as they had for fen-phen. I knew litigators very well, and I wanted no part of that.

There were other questions too. For instance, in some of our formulas, we used small doses—often only one-tenth of the amount recommended for the same ingredient when it was administered alone. How could these minuscule doses prove effective? Everything I read about sub-therapeutic doses was negative. Then there was the peculiar use of anthropomorphic descriptions in Chinese medicine, where herbs are characterized by roles such as "king" or "minister" or "assistant" or "guide." What exactly was chi, and why couldn't we pin it down? So many questions!

Like most Americans, I had always assumed that doctors knew what they were doing and that what they didn't know couldn't hurt me. My mom's experience called that assumption into question. Faced with these puzzles, I did what litigators always do when presented with new information—I dug in, trying to understand it and the forensic experts I envisioned myself deposing. I studied herbal medicine primarily from the perspective of a Western scientist, not an Eastern practitioner; the litigation experts would be scientists, not herbalists. I sought to understand the pharmacology of botanical medicine—how the drugs worked, how they interacted, and how the interactions could be beneficial rather than harmful. Along the way, I earned some patents and developed some formulas myself. I also learned to see the risks and rewards of conventional pharmacology differently.

I came to see that even from a Western perspective, the Eastern approach to medicine (small doses of many ingredients rather than big doses of one or two) made a lot more sense than the conventional Western method. I thought, no wonder we take more medicine and feel worse for it! I also grew frustrated with how the natural methods and their benefits, which I witnessed firsthand, were not broadly taught or discussed.

In 2023 I teamed up with a longtime friend Ben Bramwell to change that. I initially met Ben during my first years at RidgeCrest. He was then president of the Utah Association of Naturopathic Physicians and had succeeded in expanding prescriptive rights for naturopathic doctors (NDs) in our state.

Ben helped me understand many of the basic principles of natural medicine and how they worked in the real world. I owe much of my understanding to his teachings.

Together, we started writing a series of articles for the *Townsend Letter for Doctors*, a newsletter published by Jonathan Collins, MD, of Port Townsend, Washington, since 1983. Over forty years, Jonathan has brought cutting-edge alternative and complementary medicine ideas to light. I'm grateful that he published these ideas. I hope they will continue to find an open-minded audience.

This book has been far too long coming. We are advocating for a future that embraces traditional medicinal practices within a safer and more efficient health care framework, aiming to reduce our reliance on pharmaceuticals.

—Matt Warnock, 2024

Introduction

In general, there is a degree of doubt, caution, and modesty,

which, in all kinds of scrutiny and decision,

ought forever to accompany a just reasoner.

—David Hume

Some years ago, in an interview on National Public Radio, a doctor opined that scientists knew "about sixty percent of everything there is to know" about the human body. Shortly thereafter, researchers announced that they had just discovered what is arguably the largest organ in the body: the interstitium. Scientists previously assumed the existence of this watery space between the organs in the abdomen to be a nonentity, but a new method of microscopic slide preparation opened a new way of looking at this connective tissue that holds other organs in place, circulates extracellular fluid, affects blood pressure, and drains into the lymphatic system.[1]

In medicine especially, it pays to be humble and to be willing to put on a different set of glasses sometimes. We don't know what we don't know, but it's probably a lot more than we think we know now. Mark Twain allegedly said, "It ain't what I don't know that gets me into trouble. It's what I know for sure that just ain't so."

What Do We Really Know?

Epistemology isn't often taught in medical schools, but in scientific circles, falsifiability[2] and its relation to empirical evidence are hot topics.[3] We can positively prove very few scientific points; in science, we usually aim to disprove—not prove—a hypothesis. Our beliefs are based on varying amounts and quality of evidence, interpreted through different models and contexts, and they are always changing. Since the line between belief and knowledge is hazy and subjective, we shouldn't become too attached to what we think we know. Over two thousand years ago, Socrates famously said, "I believe that I know nothing." He may have had the right approach all along.

In daily life, however, there are many things that we take for granted. We assume the sun will rise tomorrow, that gravity will continue to operate, and that what worked yesterday will probably work today. For thousands of years, humans and animals have turned to herbal medicines to treat health complaints from abdominal pain to zygomycosis. Medicinal herbs have been found in Neanderthal teeth from twelve thousand years ago,[4] consistent with usage back to prehistoric times.[5] Until about a hundred years ago, herbs were the primary means of medical treatment, and in many parts of the world, they still are. Herbal medicines can be just as effective as modern drugs for many conditions. They are also usually safer, gentler, cheaper, more sustainable, and less polluting solutions. However, they can be variable in quality and availability, and they work better in combination than they do alone, for reasons we'll explore.

Why Don't We Use Herbs More?

Here in the United States, herbal medicine remains an obscure backwater. A handful of generic herbal drugs, most from the late nineteenth and early twentieth centuries, can only be sold in strict compliance with FDA monographs. New herbal drugs must follow the same expensive premarket approval (PMA) process used by pharmaceuticals. This isn't feasible for most natural products because they can't be patented, and the regulatory costs are unlikely to be recovered in the marketplace. For most new herbal medicines, there is simply no viable path to drug status.

As a result, most herbal medicines appear on the market as dietary supplements. These products cannot claim to "diagnose, treat, cure, or prevent any disease," even when compelling evidence supports such uses. FDA regulations forbid the mention of any diseases or symptoms in the usage directions. The regulations only allow that the product labeling speak to the support of normal body structures and functions. Making other claims leads FDA to categorize the supplement as an "unapproved new drug." This legal framework hampers innovation in herbal medicine and impedes the discussion of its scientific foundations, particularly in connection with specific product applications.

The Apples and Oranges of Conventional Medicine and Herbal Medicine

Another challenge is that the fundamental worldview of an herbal practitioner is very different from that of most modern medical professionals. As stated earlier, herbal practitioners tend to favor gentle, time-tested traditional ingredients, often combined in complex, new, and innovative ways. Most modern physicians prefer to use single, potent, and patented drugs that FDA approves, that facilities produce in a regulated manner, and that insurance plans reimburse. These modern pharmaceutical drugs often interact with other drugs and even with common foods like grapefruit and broccoli. Safety problems and recalls often occur even after FDA approval.

The once commonly prescribed weight loss combination fen-phen, for instance, caused heart valve disease due to one of its components (fenfluramine, or the use of a fenfluramine isomer known as dexfenfluramine) in about 30% of users.[6] This resulted in class action litigation that eventually included nearly 600,000 plaintiffs[7] and killed an as-yet-unknown number of Americans; one such victim was Helen Warnock, the mother of one of the coauthors of this book. The potency of conventional medicines, along with unsafe medication practices and errors, results in about six emergency room visits per 1,000 people in the United States every year, and prescription drugs are a leading cause of death worldwide.[8,9,10,11,12]

One significant distinction between conventional and herbal medicine lies in the traditional model of "one disease, one target, one drug." This model assumes that a single "magic bullet" drug can universally treat a disease and do so without side effects. Initially central to modern medicine, this concept is increasingly seen as oversimplified and incorrect. It was primarily adopted to streamline scientific research. However, the "magic bullet" approach does not apply well to many natural products, such as herbal medicines. These often feature complex chemistry and cannot be patented in the same way as single chemical drugs, limiting their commercial exploitation. Furthermore, FDA tends to categorize as many natural medicines as possible as drugs whenever it is acknowledged that they can actually be used to treat disease. This classification aims to restrict claims about their benefits, further muddling the regulatory landscape for natural and herbal medicines. Such policies complicate the ability of physicians and consumers to explore and consider natural alternatives, despite the growing recognition of their potential benefits and the limitations of the "magic bullet" model.

In contrast to the relatively recent "magic bullet" model, traditional Chinese, Ayurvedic (East Indian), and, to a lesser extent, Arabic and European herbal medicine traditions embrace combination therapy as the norm, while monotherapy is the exception. As a result of these differing approaches in formulation, modern physicians are often quite suspicious of the risk of drug-herb interactions when they encounter a new herbal medicine with multiple ingredients. They typically assume that these interactions are just as problematic as drug-drug interactions in conventional medicine. However, combinations of herbal medicines often exist because they are empirically found to reduce the risk of adverse reactions. Moreover, historically, conventional medicine has dismissed alternative medicine as primitive, unscientific, and unregulated, among other criticisms. But this attitude is gradually changing. For example, a hospital that integrates both conventional and alternative treatments provided part of Dr. Bramwell's training.

What Is Evidence?

Some physicians assert that legitimate medicine must meet the strict evidence criteria of conventional medicine, especially in the face of many natural products whose efficacy is based largely on empirical evidence, rather than the scientifically validated forms they recognize. They dismiss "complementary" or "alternative" medicine, insisting that only treatments conforming to evidence-based medicine (EBM) standards are valid. According to these physicians, any treatment not supported by such evidence does not qualify as medicine at all.[13] They adhere strictly to one framework of "evidence" as they define it and dismiss anything outside of their box as inconsequential.

A counterview would argue that it is extremely important to allow some level of flexibility as to what constitutes evidence and to remember that if we get too strict on the definition, it may be hard to put on a new set of glasses that opens our awareness—just as if we keep looking at old histology slides in the same traditional manner, we risk overlooking the interstitium as a true organ, leaving its significance forever undiscovered, unappreciated, and misunderstood.

The reality is that over thousands of years, herbal medicines have provided a wealth of empirical evidence and experience. We believe that this historical evidence, combined with basic science work identifying clear mechanisms of action associated with these medicines, should be considered competent and reliable evidence for the purpose of speaking about herbal medicines. Examples of resources that capture this empirical evidence are the materia medica of the Eclectic physicians in the early-twentieth-century United States and the Chinese pharmacopoeia. This doesn't mean that clinical trials can't offer wonderful insight. They do. However, as you will learn in this book's first chapter, today's clinical trials also have inherent limitations. When a trial does not show an expected effect of an herbal medicine, it does not follow that there is then no value in the centuries of empirical evidence collected through observation of the effects of herbal medicine in a wide, mixed, and variable population. The more we restrict our view of what evidence is valid, the more we bias our conclusions.

Allowing empirical (nonclinical trial) evidence to influence clinical decision-making is a big shift in thinking that probably makes many uncomfortable. We get that. On the other hand, even some of the best thinkers in modern EBM conclude that there is a real art in applying evidence from clinical trial populations to clinical decision-making for individual patients with unique circumstances.[14] Drawing on the experience of generations of herbal practitioners, combined with an understanding of plants' medicinal chemistry, isn't all that different—it's just supported by evidence from different sources, with their own strengths and weaknesses.

The approach of embracing empirical evidence reminds us of a *National Geographic* article from some years ago showing a reporter standing in a remote area with local villagers, within striking distance of cobras. The reporter had antivenom handy in case of being bitten, which was wise and right. But the villagers were also standing by with their traditional herbal medicines, just in case. Things don't necessarily have to be studied in clinical trials before they can be helpful, and not all clinical trials are as definitive as some seem to think.

If you are firmly attached to the "magic bullet" model and believe that randomized, double-blind, placebo-controlled trials are the only valid form of medical evidence, it's worth examining these assumptions more closely. The "magic bullet" model—the idea that one drug can universally target and treat a condition—overlooks the complex reality of human biology. Each human being is different, with different genetics (except identical twins) and also different epigenetics (how genes are expressed in a given environment), microbiome (the nonhuman cells in your skin, gut, mucosa, and respiratory systems), significant differences in what type and quantity of drug-metabolizing enzymes one's liver and other organs produce, varying medical history, environment, injuries, allergies, diet, physical fitness, mental outlook, age, beliefs, and goals.

The idea that one target and one drug could be "best" across so many variables is, frankly speaking, ludicrous.

The traditional "magic bullet" model becomes even more suspect when considering the many advantages of using multiple low doses of medicines in combination. Examples of the benefits of drug combinations include nucleoside reverse transcriptase inhibitors that are used together in lower doses to offset toxicity and increase the effectiveness of HIV treatment; combinations of lower-dose chemotherapy drugs that are less toxic and more effective when used together in treating cancer; and combinations of antihypertensive drugs in lower doses that are safer and more effective together than when used individually. We will explore why combining herbal therapies, as in many traditional approaches, makes a lot of sense.

Aside from the scientific underpinnings of the virtue of combination therapy, another reason to embrace a combination approach is that people are naturally inclined to take this approach themselves. A practitioner may want a patient only to take one medicine, thus coming closer to conditions of a clinical trial, but to respectfully paraphrase the Harvard Law of Animal Behavior: under tightly controlled experimental conditions, animals will do as they darn well please. Explaining to patients the rational reasons for including specific ingredients in their combination medicine to more fully address their unique needs helps them understand and rightly feel more comfortable with the advice given.

While the "gold standard" of a randomized, double-blind, placebo-controlled trial can be a powerful research tool, the internal validity of such a carefully constructed set of circumstances does not necessarily have external validity.[15] Internal clinical trial results from a highly controlled population don't apply to everyone in a very diverse population. Other limitations include that, in many cases, clinical trials occur over a relatively short period of time, and it may be incorrect to assume that their benefits will continue for far longer; that both experimenters and subjects may have an uncanny ability to discern whether they are given verum or placebo; and that even when a trial shows significant results, those results are not necessarily clinically relevant.[16] The first chapter of this book goes into more detail on this subject, focusing on the inherent limitations of simple randomization in small to medium-sized populations, the lack of successful blinding in most studies, and the inherent moral problems of giving a placebo to people who are sick and really need help.

The World Is Big Enough for Both
Conventional Medicine and Herbal Medicine

Herbal medicine serves crucial functions and often outshines modern medicine in certain scenarios. Similarly, modern medicine possesses capabilities that herbal remedies lack. Both have significant roles in the market and should not monopolize or receive undue government favoritism. However, regulations should not be one-size-fits-all. Risk-based regulation must consider the unique risks of each approach and implement constraints only when necessary to protect public health. Due to differing approaches, practices, ingredients, and experience, the risk factors between herbal medicines and conventional drugs vary greatly.

The advantages of conventional medicine are well-known and well-advertised. Modern medical practice has eradicated several fatal diseases and alleviated the burden of others. However, these benefits are not without cost, including the heavy toxicity burden of prescription drugs. Moreover, people often only see the disadvantages of modern medicine when they compare it with other solutions, which rarely happens when there is only one approved and lawful medical system.

We know, for example, that conventional medicine is much better at treatment than prevention, with the notable and large exception of vaccination. This deficiency is exemplified by the common statement made by many conventional physicians to "change your diet and exercise" while not having a concrete idea of what dietary changes or exercise programs would be most therapeutic. Sadly, it is rare that the effects of drugs are compared directly to the effects of a therapeutic diet as a true, stand-alone treatment option for the treatment of a disease. Yet we would be better off if that course were used routinely, except in extreme cases like cancer where intervention with drugs really is absolutely necessary, because then we could quantify a baseline of benefit from a therapeutic diet and then consider the risk/benefit ratio of added pharmacotherapy on top of that. As an example, when researchers follow that approach in individuals with heart disease, we find, not surprisingly, that aspects of a Mediterranean diet lower the risk of death in those with cardiovascular disease.[17] It is also the case that in those willing to adhere to such a diet, the addition of statins appears to have a synergistically beneficial effect. In other words, start with healthy living choices and then add to that pharmacotherapy, when needed, very judiciously.

So what are the differences between herbal and conventional medicine? Are there areas of common ground? Are there things that conventional medicine can learn from herbal medicine, and vice versa? We believe there are, and that herbal medicine includes tools that can be used effectively by doctors and patients alike, especially for incipient or chronic complaints where the biggest hammer is not always the best choice. Sadly, the current definition of a "drug" under US law makes it all but impossible for the general public to use professional-quality herbal formulas with the most complete information. This should change.

This volume will address some of these questions, primarily from the practitioner's point of view. We'll suggest ways that herbal medicine differs from conventional medicine, with both advantages and disadvantages, and why it should be taken more seriously by lawmakers, medical practitioners, and patients alike. In particular, we'll examine some of the many weaknesses that are becoming increasingly obvious in the regulatory schemes of both conventional and alternative medicine, and suggest some possible solutions. We hope this will prompt a more complete examination and discussion of these issues.

The two authors have spent the majority of their professional lives in the field of herbal medicine. Ben, a naturopathic doctor, accumulated years of experience prescribing herbs in his tenure as a physician and continues evaluating scientific research on herbal medicines and their uses, primarily for nutraceutical companies. Matt, a former attorney and litigator, is now the second-generation owner of Ridgecrest Herbals, an herbal business that has built and reformulated complex herbal remedies for the over-the-counter market for over thirty years. Matt holds two US patents on herbal formulations.

Both Ben and Matt, with their unique perspectives and backgrounds, entered the field of herbal medicine with many questions, and after many years of practice, research, and study, they still have questions and are learning every day. But their questions today are different, and based on experience, they see some things very differently than they once did. They hope to share insight, encouraging others to explore the ideas presented and, if needed, disagree based on good reason.

CHAPTER 1

The Randomized, Double-Blind, Placebo-Controlled Trial: Gold Standard or Golden Idol?

History of the Randomized, Double-Blind, Placebo-Controlled Trial: How Did We Get Here?

The history of the randomized, double-blind, placebo-controlled trial (RDBPCT) is fascinating. In 1747 James Lind described a controlled trial in which twelve sailors aboard a British naval vessel suffering from scurvy were divided into groups of two and given various options of dietary interventions. Those receiving oranges and limes made a rapid recovery, while other groups did not.[18] In 1800 John Haygarth conducted what might be considered the first placebo-controlled study by substituting wooden rods for the metallic ones commonly used to relieve rheumatism.[19] Then, a trial in 1835 with a design well ahead of its time seems to have for the first time integrated all the elements of randomization, double-blinding, and a placebo control when comparing a homeopathic remedy in water to a placebo of plain water.[20] Later, in more widely visible efforts of the 1940s, the Medical Research Council (MRC) of the UK led a study implementing double-blinding and the use of control groups to see if the compound patulin would help treat the common cold.[21] Building on the application of these principles, a truly groundbreaking and widely recognized randomized, double-blind trial was then conducted in 1948 by the MRC to investigate the use of streptomycin compared to bed rest in the treatment of tuberculosis.[22] This latter study became a well-recognized model for future randomized, controlled trials.

The Kefauver-Harris Drug Amendments of 1962 heightened the desire to implement these techniques into clinical studies in the United States, requiring FDA-approved drugs to have "substantial evidence" to establish their efficacy.[23] Specifically the amendments state: "The term 'substantial evidence' means evidence consisting of adequate and well-controlled investigations, including clinical investigations, by experts qualified by scientific training and experience to evaluate the effectiveness of the drug involved, based on which it could fairly and responsibly be concluded by such experts that the drug will have the effect it purports." Interestingly, this "definition" doesn't actually define "substantial evidence" but rather describes a process of investigation in which "the experts are to decide what kind of evidence they would like to see and then go get it."[24]

In response to the amendments and in order to assess the efficacy of drugs already on the market, FDA first relied upon the opinions of 180 conventional medical specialists of the day (The Drug Efficacy Study 1966–1969).[25] However, in 1969 the agency published a proposed rule in the Federal Register outlining which scientific principles characterized an "adequate and well-controlled clinical investigation."[26] In addition to making clear that "uncontrolled studies or partially controlled studies are not acceptable evidence to support claims of effectiveness," the regulation also highlighted defects that would lead to a study being deemed inadequately controlled, including failure to adequately define criteria for patient selection and failure to minimize investigator bias. The regulation also allowed for three possible types of control groups: a placebo control, with or without single- or double-blinding depending on the measurement system used; an active drug control; and a historical control. While the actual regulation (and more recent FDA guidance[27]) allowed flexibility in the type of control used and whether to implement double-blinding, it marked the beginning of controlled trials as the basis to demonstrate efficacy for drug approval.

In its current form, found in 21 CFR 314.126(a), the regulation serves to guide researchers to distinguish between the effects of drugs and other influences, including "spontaneous change in the course of the disease, placebo effect, or biased observation."[28] Over time, the inclusion of randomization to facilitate comparability and the use of double-blinding and placebo controls to minimize bias has become the construct for clinical trials that, by convention, is recognized as the "gold standard" for clinical studies.[29] In practical terms, an analysis of studies used as the basis for drug approval between 2005 and 2012 found that about 89% of studies used for approval were randomized, around 79% were double-blind, and about 55% were placebo-controlled (with close to 32% using active comparator groups).[30]

Weaknesses of the RDBPCT

Experts often highlight the strengths of the RDBPCT; however, it is vital in science to challenge assumptions so that we do not become servants to them. One can appreciate the real-world weaknesses of RDBPCTs by assessing the inherent limitations of each element: randomization, double-blinding, and placebo control.

The transformative idea of randomization was clearly articulated and championed by renowned statistician R. A. Fisher while working with agricultural samples. The hope of randomization is that confounding variables can be evenly distributed between groups, allowing for greater comparability across groups. In the words of Fisher, randomization was the process "by which the validity of the test of significance may be guaranteed against corruption by the causes of disturbance which have not been eliminated."[31] With so many hidden variables in the complex human body, can we trust that simple randomization evenly distributes confounding variables?

In recent years, some have argued that in small to moderate studies, which are the mainstay of clinical research, it really doesn't.[32] In fact, one team, after reanalyzing published data from two large, multicenter trials with random replicated samples of varying size, found that simple randomization would reliably remove random differences in baseline characteristics between groups when including at least 1,000 subjects.[33] In other words, randomization would only likely protect against bias if 1,000 or more subjects were enrolled. Below this large number of subjects, "baseline characteristics were imbalanced, and substantial mean squared error in effects measurement was observed." Large numbers are thus needed for randomization to achieve its desired and assumed effect reliably. In response to this finding, some have argued that balance is not necessary because corrections can be made in statistical analysis to produce meaningful confidence intervals that allow interpretation of the data.[34] However, others persuade us that balance is, in fact, relevant because it is a means to produce results with the highest precision and least amount of bias possible.[35] The clinician, who in the real world is the client of the professional researcher, benefits from a like-for-like comparison with high precision and low bias when making decisions for a patient's care.

At first blush, blinding seems an excellent way to reduce bias in an experiment. However, relatively few studies clearly describe their methods of blinding. In some cases, due to the obvious effects of a drug in a trial, or its look, taste, or smell, doctors and participants can often accurately guess whether they're getting a placebo or the actual drug. A review of 1,599 studies characterized as blinded revealed that merely thirty-one of them assessed the effectiveness of their blinding, with successful blinding achieved approximately 45% of the time.[36] However, even in cases where blinding succeeds in accomplishing what it sets out to do, it succeeds in reducing bias only *within the experiment*. Beyond first knowing whether or not blinding took place, the problem remains of translating successfully blinded experimental results to real-world situations. Clinical practice does not occur within the confines of a blinded experiment, and how physicians interact with patients, either positively or negatively, impacts outcomes.

Using the term "iatrotherapy" to describe the effect of the physician on the healing of the patient, a thoughtful physician from some years ago stated: "A dose of enthusiastic iatrotherapy given in conjunction with an ineffectual drug will usually make patients feel better than a moderately effective drug delivered with little or no iatrotherapy."[37] By the same token, a negative bedside manner may have a bigger effect on the patient than either the verum or placebo delivered with it.

We will next delve into the significant challenge posed by the placebo component in RDBPCTs, as evidenced by historical examples.

Hindsight: Learning from Society's Wrestle with the Gold Standard: The Field Trial of the Salk Polio Vaccine

A large-scale societal reckoning with the RDBPCT came with the field trial of Jonas Salk's vaccine for poliomyelitis in 1954. The push to field trials began after Salk reported initial promising results in several hundred subjects. The investigation's ultimate structure included an RDBPCT (hereafter referred to as the placebo-controlled trial) and a unique observation study. The shaping of this design came from the interests and opinions of research scientists; the needs of the March of Dimes Foundation (The National Foundation for Infantile Paralysis), which funded the work through private donations; and the citizenry at large, which was motivated and engaged in a large-scale effort to end the scourge of polio. As persuasively argued by Meldrum,[38] this conglomeration of competing needs and groups of people is one example demonstrating that the randomized, controlled trial "is not a methodical black box but a social exercise in problem-solving." At the center of the cauldron of this particular mix of interests and people was a lay foundation that needed to demonstrate tangible progress to its donors; that is, contributions were moving the work forward to a successful conclusion. The foundation also required public involvement and endorsement from the scientific community to ensure the legitimacy of its results.

It is important to note that while the structure of the placebo-controlled trial would give the results greater validity in the eyes of many researchers, the approach prompted concern on several levels for those involved—concerns that remain relevant to the RDBPCT structure today. For example, how to handle the logistics and expenses of such a complicated protocol were of great concern to the investigators of the field trial, and these challenges are still inherent in trials of complex design today, albeit to a lesser degree. However, the most painful concern was the moral issue that still plagues placebo-controlled trials: many families who wanted access to a possibly effective intervention right away would initially receive an injection with only a placebo, with some in the placebo group being possibly unnecessarily stricken with the disease. In contrast, Salk had initially envisioned an observation trial in multiple countries that involved inoculating 388,800 children; the incidence of ensuing polio would then be compared mathematically to that of about three million unvaccinated children in those countries.[39]

In the end, the field trial included both a large placebo-controlled trial and an observation study in which second-graders at participating sites received vaccination. At the same time, observers simply watched the first- and third-graders, who received no intervention. The public more generally favored the latter approach at the time, as is evidenced by the fact that over thirty states opted for inclusion in the observation study while eleven committed to the placebo control.[40]

The urgency of the ethical concern, combined with doubts about effectively implementing the placebo-controlled trial, temporarily heightened the emotions of the usually reserved Salk as he wrote an eloquent and poignant letter to Basil O'Connor, then president of the March of Dimes Foundation:[41] "If we are aware of the fact that the presence of antibody is effective in preventing the experimental disease in animals and in man, then what moral justification can there be for intentionally injecting children with salt solution or some other placebo for the purpose of determining whether or not a procedure that produces antibody formation is effective."

This remains a powerful argument against the use of placebos. In the context of clear understanding of the pathology of disease and mechanisms by which suffering may be alleviated, what business do we really have administering placebos that presumably don't have any effect in activating necessary mechanisms in order to relieve suffering?

Salk continued: "The use of a placebo control, I am afraid, is a fetish of orthodoxy and would serve to create a 'beautiful epidemiologic' experiment over which the epidemiologist could become quite ecstatic but would make the humanitarian shudder and Hippocrates turn over in his grave."

Perhaps few scientists before or after have enjoyed Jonas Salk's aptitude for both scientific excellence and prose as he continued by laying bare the position of those who would only accept as valid results coming from an RDBPCT: "It is not a question of science, or of ethics, or of morality, upon which those who maintain the contrary position make their stand, but rather because of false pride based on values in which the worship of science involves the sacrifice of humanitarian principles on the altar of rigid methodology…in my opinion, there is no choice but to follow a course based upon the principle: 'Do unto others as you would have others do unto you.'"

Simply put, if you were facing the prospect of a terrible disease, would you rather get an intervention that might help you or a placebo? If we refuse to acknowledge the obvious answer and put placebos before patients in our research approach, haven't we sacrificed our humanity for a false pride? Should an alluring glow of acceptance from others and the glitter of self-ordained scientific authority be purchased with human suffering?

Though more weight was certainly given to data from the placebo-controlled trial, we would argue that the results of both the observation study and the placebo-controlled trial capably demonstrated a robust effect of the vaccine used. Data to this point, taken from table 3 of the published evaluation of the field trial, is shown below:[42]

Summary of results, Incidence of Paralytic Poliomyelitis in the Salk Vaccine Field Trial

	Placebo-controlled trial		Observation study	
	Vaccinated	Placebo	Vaccinated	Control
N	200,745	201,229	221,998	725,173
Cases of paralytic poliomyelitis	33	115	38	330
Rate of paralytic polio cases	16/100,000	57/100,000	17/100,000	46/100,000

Moreover, as represented in table 7 from the same publication (Francis 1955), the vaccine caused a significant reduction in the rate of paralytic polio in both studies, whether compared to placebo or to observed control, with a p value < 0.001 in both comparisons. Thus, the results of both the placebo-controlled and observation trials show the vaccine reduces the rate of paralytic polio.

While in this case there could be discussion as to which study better represented the true rate of vaccine effectiveness, a large effect is obvious in both studies. This prompts an important and interesting question: if placebo had not been given, and if instead vaccine had been injected in its place in an even larger observation study, how would the world have reacted to the results? Based on the collected observation data, it is hard to argue that had this hinge of scientific history swung solely on observational data rather than on data from a placebo-controlled trial, the benefit would have been anything but obvious. Most of the public would have demanded access to the vaccine, and the rate of paralytic polio would still have plummeted.

This leads to the next important question: Was it really necessary to subject children and their families to the risk (and in some cases, the horrific reality) of preventable disease by using a placebo instead of a vaccine? How much false hope, deception, and unnecessary suffering is enough to appease the demands of the scientific idol that is widely worshipped as the "gold standard"?

When the Gold Standard Doesn't Fit: The NCI Approach

When a gold standard of research structure exists, there is a strong desire to conform research methods to that standard. This is understandable on several levels, both because researchers naturally desire to do the best work possible by using the best tools available and because work that conforms to a gold standard is more likely to be accepted. Nevertheless, we can learn a lot by asking where the use of the gold standard becomes most problematic and why.

One of the domains in which the gold standard of RDBPCTs faces significant challenges is in the development of new cancer drugs. This is one of the areas of clinical care where physicians face the reality of working with extremely ill, vulnerable, and dying patients desperate to try new treatments that might either cure their cancer or at least prolong their lives. In this context, the moral issue of placebo use is magnified because someone may be denied access to a drug that ends up not only reducing morbidity but being the difference between life and death.

In response to the patient need, the National Cancer Institute (NCI) developed a system for the distribution of experimental drugs that showed promise in animal models to then be tried in a relatively small clinical setting, before moving on to progressively larger stages of study if a drug showed potential. NCI was roundly criticized for this approach in a series of articles in the *Washington Post* in the early 1980s:[43] a former NCI official, Vincent Bono, stated that the program was like "donating someone's body to science while they are still alive," and Robert Young of FDA compared the NCI's approach to generals in Vietnam with the attitude that "we've got to burn the village to save it."

During a congressional hearing sparked by the controversy,[44] NCI's director at the time, Vincent DeVita, firmly supported NCI's method of providing and testing experimental drugs to try and meet patient needs. He highlighted that the *Washington Post* articles mistakenly attributed many deaths to the experimental drugs, when in reality, the patients' underlying burden of disease was the actual cause of death. He also highlighted that the research was contributing to progress in the treatment of cancer, with an improvement to 45% of cancers being curable at that time. Importantly, Dr. DeVita explained that NCI's approach was based on the need to do something for the patient, to innovate for the patient's benefit in spite of practical market obstacles, such as the development of a new drug at that time taking ten to fifteen years and thirty to forty million dollars.

In emphatic defense of NCI's approach, he stated: "There are risks associated with early drug testing but the most serious toxicity of all is the unnecessary death from cancer....Cancer drugs must be tested for ethical reasons in patients with the most advanced forms of the disease who have exhausted all available treatment....Any system of drug distribution we develop that denies any cancer patient access to these resources is wrong."

The approach fostered by NCI had a different emphasis than that of typical efforts overseen by FDA. Part of this was evidenced in the fact that whereas early Phase I trials for drugs used to treat other diseases typically focus on toxicity and understanding a drug's pharmacology in the human body, the early trials in the NCI approach included efficacy as an objective because of the pressing need to provide the patient with treatment options. Understanding toxicity was also a concern, but these substances were already known to be toxic prior to testing in humans. The approach framed by NCI, while not reliant on the RDBPCT, was responsive to pressing patient demand and had already helped to improve patient outcomes. As of this writing, NCI's website explains that while placebos can be a way of reducing bias, they are rarely used in trials of cancer treatments. Currently, for example, placebos are used when there is not an existing standard of treatment that has proven to be of benefit.[45]

Some would argue that the NCI approach clearly makes sense in the case of very sick cancer patients when the issue of placebo is so clearly problematic but that the RDBPCT should still be the gold standard in other less dire clinical circumstances. However, given the increasing understanding of limitations inherent in randomization when used in smaller and medium-sized studies and the blinding reviewed above, we are unconvinced with this argument. It also seems to us that those who are willing to accept the moral drawbacks of a placebo in one condition but not another are on slippery ground: when does the level of suffering of one patient permit the deception of a placebo and the level of suffering of another patient not lead to its use? Our concerns increase as we consider how well-designed cohort studies are generally viable for estimating therapeutic effects and understanding safety, as reviewed below.

The RDBPCT versus Observation Studies

One of the realizations shared above is that the Salk vaccine field trials showed similar estimates of efficacy in both the placebo-controlled trial and the completed observation study. Work in more recent decades confirms that on average meta-analysis of randomized controlled trials with many subjects and well-done observation studies do lead to very similar estimates of efficacy,[46,47] despite assertions to the contrary. Additionally, real-world observation studies that include larger groups over longer periods provide greater opportunity to understand the toxicity of an intervention compared to randomized, controlled trials often constructed to show efficacy in the short to medium term. While drugs are often approved based on studies done over a few years, it may take five or more years for the full picture of a drug's toxicity to become appreciated.[48] A good example of this is the increased risk of myocardial infarction seen in patients using protease inhibitor drugs, an effect that only became apparent over six years and was found during the course of an observational trial after the drugs were already on the market.[49]

In order to construct observation trials with the most helpful design possible, others have pointed out that observational studies utilizing a cohort design, which collect data longitudinally and thus preserve the relationship between exposure and outcome (temporality), provide a higher level of evidence of causality. This is in contrast to case-control studies that identify outcomes and then search for previous exposure.[50] Therefore, data from observation studies with a cohort design may be more valuable. When the source is large, even national, registries or databases, high quality and informative data can be collected to inform decision-making. While such observational data currently seems to fit the category of real-world data (RWD) that FDA suggests should be used as confirmatory evidence in addition to data obtained from controlled trials,[51] we would suggest, based on the literature reviewed above, that high-quality observational data should be viewed as more than just confirmatory.

Conclusion

It is important to acknowledge that no study design is perfect and free of risk. Every design can face issues such as confounding from unknown variables, bias, or difficulty in separating the signal that represents a treatment's effect from the noise of spontaneous changes seen during the course of living or the progress of disease.

However, as we have pointed out above, simple randomization in small and medium-size trials may not offer the level of protection against confounding that it was previously believed to. Blinding methods certainly have value in removing bias during a study, but they are often not employed effectively. Moreover, blinded conditions are simply not consistent with the circumstances of actual clinical care, highlighting some limits of applicability from the trials of today and the use of an intervention in the wider world. And placebo controls are morally challenged, especially but not exclusively in the case of the most severe diseases, when a patient deserves every chance of real or potential help.

In short, the principal problem with the RDBPCT as a gold standard is that, in practical use, the beautiful scientific idea has real-world limitations in how randomization and blinding are done and inherent moral liability. Simply because a trial is randomized, double-blind, and placebo-controlled does not mean it is exempt from pitfalls that lead to a high number of research claims turning out to be false.[52] Moreover, while large studies generally offer more protection against false findings, the perceived need for elements of randomization, blinding, and placebo control should be seen as diminished when the actual effect of an intervention is very large and obvious. After all, a group of only two subjects was needed to show that eating citrus fruit was a cure for scurvy, and the obvious effect of Salk's polio vaccine was evident in both observation and placebo-controlled studies.

Further, there are other alternatives in study design to consider. Well-done observation studies can generally estimate the effect of an intervention. They represent understanding obtained within the flow of clinical care and thus have wide applicability. They are free of the moral drawbacks of administering placebos that provide false hope to sick patients who really deserve the best shot at therapeutic intervention. In addition, such studies can provide a more complete view of an intervention's safety profile, which manifests fully only over time. Finally, an important question to consider is this: If randomization doesn't work as effectively as believed in small to medium studies, and if blinding often fails, is there really much effectual difference between many RDBPCTs and observation studies? Based on our review, we conclude that well-done observation studies, especially those that use prospective cohorts and clinical registries/databases with large amounts of data, should be embraced much more enthusiastically for clinical evaluation.

If we continue to regard the RDBPCT as the unquestionable gold standard, ignoring its practical and moral flaws, and dismiss legitimate alternatives as inferior, what consequences might arise for scientific progress and patient care? In this case, we are not merely employing a tool: we have unwittingly fallen into the worship of an idol of our own making, and we will find ourselves unquestioningly sacrificing to it.

As we move forward, we'll delve into the implications of a drug marketplace dominated by products approved primarily using the current "gold standard."

CHAPTER 2

The Danger of Using Drugs as Directed

One of the world's most frustrating and heartbreaking realities is that patients can get very sick from using many kinds of medicine, and pharmaceutical drugs in particular, for therapeutic purposes. A recent national estimate based on NEISS-CADES data for 2017 to 2019 is that medication harm results in 6.1 (95% CI, 4.8–7.5) emergency room (ER) visits per 1,000 people in the US population annually. Moreover, about two-thirds of the time [69.1% (95% CI, 63.6%–74.7%)], these visits result from either the proper use of medication or patients trying to use the medication as directed but making unintentional errors.[53] Based on the US Census Bureau's population estimate of the national population from early April 2023 (334,571,431 for April 3),[54] and assuming the rates above haven't changed drastically in just the last few years, this indicates the United States could expect on the order of 1.4 million ER visits in 2023 just from people trying to use medicines as directed.

Medicines Most Frequently Implicated and Their Long-Term Effects

Which medicines are most frequently implicated in contributing to an ER visit when used therapeutically? Overall, anticoagulants account for about 21.5% (95% CI 16.5–26.4), making it the category of medicines with the highest such rate (Budnitz 2021). As one might anticipate, the primary contributor to these cases is often warfarin (accounting for 12.1% of ER visits with harm from medicines used therapeutically [95% CI 9.7–14.5]), but newer direct-acting anticoagulants also account for a sizeable incidence of such events, estimated at 8.5% (CI 5.9–11.2).

Surprisingly, newer anticoagulation drugs may only improve safety a little. Diabetic agents (led by insulin) come in next, accounting for 13.7% (95% 11.8–15.6) of visits, while antibiotics account for 12.8% (95% CI 10.8–14.9) of these unfortunate occurrences and analgesics 6.6% (5.7–7.5). The rate for analgesics is driven mainly by prescription opioids. People over forty-five visit the ER much more frequently due to their use of anticoagulants and diabetic agents. Meanwhile, antibiotics most often create issues for patients under five years old (Budnitz 2021).

These data show that medications, even when administered carefully, have inherently exaggerated risks in clinically sensitive situations such as regulating coagulation, managing swings in blood sugar, and treating bacterial infections. In contrast, herbal and homeopathic medicines together accounted for about 1.1% (0.9–1.4) of such events, while vitamin and mineral products accounted for approximately 0.9% (0.8–1.0).

Of course, while data from ER visits provide insight as to when medications are associated with serious acute adverse events, we must consider that these data do not capture every adverse event related to therapeutic drug use. Patients are treated for drug-induced adverse effects in other clinical settings, and it is probably not true that every case of a drug-induced adverse event is clearly recognized as such, perhaps especially when an individual has consumed a drug for an extended period of time. For example, cardiovascular events caused by long-term use of NSAIDs may be diagnosed and treated as a cardiovascular event without the clinicians providing immediate care ever connecting the event clearly with previous long-term NSAID use. Considering the widespread use of NSAIDs, we will specifically highlight the associated risks of these drugs in the following section.

The major toxicities of nonaspirin NSAIDs include cardiovascular events, kidney dysfunction, and damage to the gastrointestinal tract that can include severe bleeding. Reflective of this, in a post-hoc analysis of an RDBPCT (the PRECISION trial) of 24,081 subjects (mean age 63.2+/-9.4 years, mean treatment duration 20.3+/-16.0 months, mean follow-up of 34.1+/-13.4 months) with arthritis and moderate to high cardiovascular risk given a daily NSAID (ibuprofen 600 mg TID, naproxen 375 mg BID, or celecoxib 100 mg BID) plus a proton pump inhibitor, approximately one in twenty subjects experienced such a major toxicity over one to two years of use.[55] With particular regard to adverse effects on the kidney, the results indicated significant declines in kidney filtration rates among those who started the study with normal baseline rates. Specifically, a greater-than-30% decrease occurred in 13.8% of the ibuprofen group, 9.8% of the naproxen group, and 8.7% of the celecoxib group—the last being significantly lower than the other two groups.[56]

In a more general population represented in the Women's Health Initiative,[57] of 160,801 participants (mean follow-up 11.2 years), 53,142 reported some period of regular NSAID use (at least twice a week) during data collection. The hazard ratio (HR, a ratio of how often a hazardous event occurs in two groups being compared) for an adverse cardiovascular outcome in those with regular use of selective COX-2 inhibitors (celecoxib and rofecoxib) versus those with no regular NSAID use was 1.13 (95% CI 1.04–1.23), while in those taking NSAIDs with more COX-2 inhibition than COX-1 inhibition (primarily naproxen), the HR was 1.17 (95% CI 1.10–1.24). The hazard ratio for those taking an NSAID (primarily ibuprofen) with more COX-1 than COX-2 inhibition did not significantly increase (1.01, 95% CI 0.95–1.07).

The effects of older NSAIDs, such as indomethacin, on the upper gastrointestinal (GI) tract have been known for decades, with increased gastric and duodenal ulcerations and mucosal erosions reported.[58] While health care professionals have valued NSAIDs with selective COX-2 inhibition due to reported lower rates of GI damage,[59] there are some findings in populations with longer-term use suggesting a lack of protective effect, specifically in the small bowel, with selective COX-2 inhibition.[60,61] Moreover, it should be pointed out that the common practice of combining a COX-2 inhibitor with a proton pump inhibitor may essentially negate any benefit of selective COX-2 inhibitors in decreasing small bowel damage.[62]

In addition to these significant toxicities, NSAIDs are also rarely associated with a reaction from the body's immune system, causing a non-infectious form of meningitis that, among other symptoms, results in hearing loss that is likely reversible after discontinuation of the drug.[63]

Opioid Risks and the Current Epidemic

Given the current opioid epidemic, some focus on the risks of the therapeutic use of opioids is also merited here, with the first concern being how likely it is that therapeutic use of prescription opioids will lead to opioid abuse, adding to the current opioid crisis.

This is a difficult question to answer. The available data indicate that the likelihood of issues arising from therapeutic opioid use is influenced by the duration of use and the dose of morphine equivalents administered.[64] A helpful study by Edlund analyzed data from 197,269 subjects who received opioid prescriptions following a new diagnosis of chronic, non-cancer pain. In this study, length of use had a greater impact on risk than actual dose, though the combination of chronic use and high dose produced the greatest rate of problematic use. The rate of those developing an opioid-use disorder was 6.1% (23/378) in those exposed to both a chronic and high dose use pattern. The risk was much lower for those given acute, high doses, at 0.12% (15/12,378). Rates for other dose patterns were 1.28% (47/3,654) for chronic, medium dose; 0.12% (101/83,542) for acute, medium dose; 0.72% (50/6,902) for chronic, low dose; and 0.12% (111/90,415) acute, low dose. The predominance of acute dosing patterns by prescribers in this population may well have prevented many cases of opioid use disorder.

While the above data help with understanding the risk of incident opioid use disorders in those beginning opioid treatment, it is also helpful to consider data related to those with an established long-term pattern of use in the context of chronic pain and mental health symptoms, particularly depression and anxiety. Banta-Green reports insightful work in this regard,[65] based on interviews with 704 patients with non-cancer chronic pain in an integrated group medical practice. These patients had an average total days' supply of opioids of 349 (SD 241) in the previous 365 days and an average opioid dose in morphine equivalents of 50 mg (SD 64). Opioid dependence was present in 13% of the patients, while opioid abuse without dependence was present in an additional 8%.

One could describe the population as falling into three different groups: a typical group of the majority with persistent, moderate mental health (depression, anxiety) and pain symptoms; an addictive behaviors group with increased mental health symptoms and opioid problems but with pain levels similar to those in the typical group; and a pain dysfunction group that had significantly higher pain, mental health, and opioid problems. The prescribed average daily opioid dose was three times higher in the two latter groups than in the typical group.

Additional work by Boscarino in outpatients with non-cancer pain and chronic opioid use found that the factors of depression, psychotropic medication use, pain impairment, and age under sixty-five years could predict the risk of current dependence,[66] a rate that may have been as high as 26% in their population.

In order to mitigate the risks of prescription opioids, careful consideration of the patient's mental health profile seems central. While physicians should consistently initiate these conversations, informed patients also help themselves by alerting prescribers to mental health issues that need to be considered before prescription decisions about opioid medications are made.

Prescription Errors and Their Impact

While the above information focuses primarily on the dangers of therapeutic use of prescription medications, it is also important to review the dangers that can arise when making errors in a drug prescription. It is quite challenging to clarify the scope of prescription errors, at least in outpatient settings. One recent review of prescription errors in the primary care setting found that estimates of inappropriately prescribed medications ranged from as low as 0.19% in some studies to 98.2% in others.[67]

One of the challenges in interpreting these data is that most studies on the topic use their own definition of what actually constitutes an error. It might be more informative to look at prescription error rates in the ER, where they occur most commonly, likely due to the stress of the environment. In fact, one relatively recent study found that errors in prescriptions given to patients as they leave the ER happen at a rate of about 16.5%.[68] In another study, errors in the prescription of anti-coagulants for patients leaving the ER, specifically, were found to occur at a rate of around 40%, with significantly more errors by currently in-training residents.[69]

Fortunately, the extent to which prescription errors lead to adverse events varies. In fact, the majority of these errors are relatively minor. This might include errors like a pharmacist dispensing an incorrect quantity of the correct dosage or giving an inappropriate number of refills. Nonetheless, errors can, of course, cause tragic adverse events. In the case of the anticoagulant study cited (Gregory 2020), prescription errors led to readmission of a patient in 0.6% of cases, while another ER study in France found that ER prescription errors led to serious consequences about 14% of the time; importantly, having a pharmacist review prescriptions could substantially reduce the rate.[70]

This brings us to potential solutions for reducing prescription errors. Double-checks of prescriptions by pharmacists are undoubtedly one of the best ways to reduce prescription error rates in just about any clinical setting.[71,72,73] An ongoing feedback system that alerts prescribers about identified errors also helps reduce future mistakes.[74] Not surprisingly, there is evidence that an effective way to reduce errors in medical prescriptions is to utilize electronic prescription systems instead of having any handwritten orders that need to be transcribed.[75] Many prescribing providers and their institutions are actively implementing these types of changes.

We also advocate here for patients to become politely proactive in reviewing prescriptions with prescribers. In all but the most hurried circumstances, a good form of communication initiated by the patient might include: "So, to review, you are prescribing me a drug named ____ to treat my ____. How much is in each dose, and how often am I supposed to take it?" The vast majority of practitioners are competent, but that doesn't mean it isn't helpful to have patients actively engaged in the process of their own care, making sure they respectfully allow the prescriber (whether the prescriber takes advantage of it or not) to verbally review specifics of a prescription before the patient has it filled. We are all human. Reflective communication by the patient, combined with other approaches already shown to reduce errors, such as pharmacist review, electronic prescription, and a prescriber feedback system, seems to be a multipronged approach worth implementing.

While pharmacotherapy is ingrained in modern life, and can be life-saving and life-improving, there are significant risks and damage inherent to its use. The use of anticoagulants, diabetic drugs, antibiotics, and analgesics seems to carry the greatest risks. Amid the current opioid epidemic, data emphasize the need to minimize both the duration and dosage of opioid use whenever possible while also considering risk factors for abuse, such as depression and anxiety. Pharmacist review of prescriptions can help reduce prescription errors. Other interventions, such as the use of electronic prescription systems and prescriber feedback systems, as well as patients and providers simply taking the time to review the specifics of a prescription together during the clinical encounter, can also help reduce prescription errors so that drug use is as safe as possible.

If these early chapters have led you to question the current state of medical research, drug approval, and drug administration, know we share your concerns. But the risks of prescription drug use also lead us to value the importance of understanding how drugs (natural or synthetic) work in the body, which we discuss in the next several chapters. Further, we will show you how traditional formulation and delivery of herbal medicines can provide advantages, providing efficacy without sacrificing safety.

CHAPTER 3

Drug Receptor Theory

Receptor Theory and Drug Effects

Since we are exploring the effects of drugs in considerable detail in this book, it is important to understand the theory underpinning the understanding of drugs' powerful effects on the human body. For many years, their mechanisms of action were mostly unknown. In many cases, they still are. However, receptor theory has proved helpful in describing and predicting how many drugs work, whether we know all the specifics or not.

History of Receptor Theory: The Nuts and Bolts

Near the beginning of the twentieth century, researchers suggested that drugs (ligands) interacted with some kind of receptors in the human body to create drug effects. This idea gained traction and evidence by the middle of the century.[76,77]

Ligands bind to receptors on the surface of specific cells. The binding strength, affinity, and duration can vary, resulting in either the receptor's activation or inactivation. When ligand binding leads to activation, it can in turn lead to either an increase or decrease in a cellular function[78] by modulating electrical activity or chemical messaging either within or outside the cell. Ligands that activate the receptor to induce a drug's effect are called agonists, and ligands that prevent receptor activation are known as antagonists. Several variations exist in mechanisms of receptor agonism and antagonism, but this is the basic idea.

In the years following the development of receptor theory, researchers have accumulated substantial evidence (such as from scanning electron microscopes) to show that the theory is mostly correct. However, even before that evidence accumulated, it provided a helpful explanation of the action of many drugs, even when detailed information about specific cells and receptors was lacking.

Drug Agonists and Antagonists

Opioids are just one example of drug agonists. Researchers realized early on that receptors in the body responded to various opioid alkaloids, including morphine, heroin (originally a Bayer drug), codeine, and others. These receptors are known to bind with endogenous opioids, internally generated peptides including endorphins, which our bodies naturally produce to ease pain. The brain produces endorphins in "fight or flight" situations to kill pain, increase endurance, and permit escape from life-threatening situations. Why did certain plants develop the ability to trigger these same opioid receptors? We don't know for sure, but it is clear humans have been using these agonists for thousands of years as analgesics (painkillers) and for other perceived benefits. (It's interesting that we often associate opioid receptors mainly with synthetic alkaloids, even though their primary function is to interact with the body's naturally occurring opioid peptides. It might actually have been better to call these the endorphin receptors.) On the other hand, an example of a drug antagonist is naloxone, a drug that also binds to opioid receptors but blocks and can reverse the effects of opioid agonists.

Under receptor theory, the effect and duration of a drug are determined by several factors, including:

- The chemical nature of the ligand (drug molecule)
- The target cell and receptor, and the cellular action it modulates
- How many ligands are available for binding
- How easily and strongly ligands bind to the target receptors
- Whether other, nontarget receptors will bind to the same ligands
- Whether other, competing ligands will bind to the same receptors
- The fraction of total receptors bound at any given time

- How long ligands stay bound to the receptor
- How receptors become unbound
- How fast enzymes in the GI tract, liver, kidneys, and other organs make them ready to be excreted from the body

Receptor Theory in Clinical Practice

Receptor theory assumes that an equation can describe the relationship between drug concentrations and biological response over a short period. Thus, a pharmacological effect can be produced and maintained by getting the right dose and frequency of drug administration to meet clinical goals. Clinicians may use a "titration for effect" strategy, adjusting the dose until they achieve the desired effects with minimal adverse effects. But this is time-consuming, so it's often the exception, not the rule, in prescribing.[79,80] Instead, many clinicians use a "standard dose," based on body weight (see Robinson 2014 for an example of this in a neonate population[81]), or, as is increasingly the case with chemotherapy drugs, a dose is selected from a range of commonly available dosages based on predefined ranges of body surface area in an approach called "dose banding."[82,83] Even the "one-size-fits-all" fixed-dose approach is still common: "Take two aspirin and call me in the morning" may be used regardless of the gender, weight, age, or condition of the patient.

Individual Considerations

There is nothing in receptor theory to suggest that all individuals will have the same magnitude of response to any given drug. In fact, all of the available evidence points to the opposite conclusion: many variables are in play at any given time, and most will change over time. Statistics teaches us that while there may be a central tendency to our drug response data, there will always be individual variations and outliers will always occur. Given enough data, we can predict roughly how many outliers there will be. However, absent very clear foresight based on genetic predispositions, we can't currently predict who they will be or how far they will fall from the normal response.

So no matter how much population data we collect, we can never really answer the two top-most questions in every patient's mind: "will this drug work for me?" and "will I have an adverse reaction?" Statistics allow us to make inferences about larger populations from smaller groups, but it doesn't work in the opposite direction—statistics don't predict individual results. If you experience a particularly nasty adverse event, then rates for others don't matter: your rate is effectively 100%. Only hindsight is twenty-twenty.

Most studies of how a drug moves through the body (pharmaco-kinetics) and its resulting effects (pharmacodynamics) are done in the short term, even when using drugs over a much longer term. One of the aspects of prescription drug use that only becomes clear over a long time and with lots of doses (perhaps a billion) is a drug's toxicology, or adverse events and reactions caused by drugs. Toxic effects can be grouped generally in several different ways (depending on what source you read), such as:

- Subtle effects, which are hard to detect, easily tolerated, and don't interfere with compliance to treatment
- Nuisance effects, which are more noticeable and may interfere with taking the drug
- Severe effects, which result in hospitalization, death, or permanent injury or require medical treatment to prevent these outcomes

However, these categories don't come with built-in, easily recognized boundaries. Subtle, even unnoticeable effects can be the tip of the spear for permanent injury or even fatal reactions later on; other adverse effects may manifest with continued exposure or culminate only when exposures exceed a certain threshold that the body can effectively clear. The old story of Mithridates[84] illustrates how the body may be able to clear some poisons more effectively after continued exposure, making adverse effect characterization a moving target. A likely more informative approach would be to plot toxicity data based on the percentage of the population that experiences each adverse effect over a range of doses (in what is known as a quantal response curve). Still, effects often differ from patient to patient, and it may be difficult to detect adverse effects from random, unrelated health concerns before a drug is approved. There is an old joke in the drug industry that a drug executive, on hearing that FDA approved a new drug, quipped, "Now the real testing begins!"

Over longer periods of time, the body tends to adapt to drug effects in many ways, including the following:

- Generally, the body tends to return to homeostasis, adjusting itself to compensate for new conditions, including drug intake.
- The body may generate more or fewer receptor cells, change the time that a receptor stays intact, and even change the response in the cell that occurs with receptor binding, all of which can change the patient's relative sensitivity to the drug.[85]
- A patient may develop an allergy to a particular drug; some allergies are more common than others.
- In many cases, drugs may disrupt or weaken the body's self-regulatory mechanisms.

Here are just two examples:
- Endorphins are some of the opioid peptides naturally released when the body needs pain control. When the body receives opioid alkaloid painkillers, however, the natural release of endorphins is inhibited.[86,87] This doesn't mean that prescription opioids are never needed, but inhibition of our body's natural pain-relieving system is another factor to consider.
- Thyroid hormones (T3/T4) decrease production of TSH, which in turn further reduces the natural production of thyroid

hormones. While lifelong administration of thyroid hormone may be needed, there is some evidence that about 30% of patients with mild (non-overt) hypothyroidism can resume their natural pattern of thyroid hormone secretion.[88]

Receptor Theory and Herbal Medicine

Receptor theory has proved useful over many years, and there is no reason to believe that it isn't as useful in herbal medicine as it is in pharmacology, though there are some important differences too. For example, conventional pharmacology usually deals with the effect of a single drug, while the maelstrom of human physiological processes swirls around it. Those processes include sleeping, waking, eating, digestion, elimination, exertion, rest, and all the other human activities. On the other hand, herbal medicine doesn't deal with a single active compound like conventional drugs.

Consider as an example the humble mint (*Mentha*). There are dozens of mint species[89] and hundreds of hybrids and cultivars. While the aromatic essential oil may be up to 80% menthol, the active constituents of several species used medicinally vary greatly by location and season,[90] perhaps even more than by species, and may also include menthone, carvone, limonene, and many other physiologically active terpenes. Garlic has over 200 identified constituent compounds.[91] In addition to helping the plant species survive and be able to reproduce (for example, aromatic plants like mint may ward off deer[92]), a plant's many phytochemicals can have immense benefits to humans, such as the blood pressure lowering effects of garlic[93] and the antispasmodic effects of some mints, notably peppermint.[94] Indeed, plants have many medicinal properties that encourage their collection, use, distribution, and cultivation.

Variability of content is one of the inherent realities of herbal medicine, and it makes the application of receptor theory less straightforward because in the case of these medicines, more chemicals are dancing with different receptors at the same time. Conventional medicine might view such complexity and variability with concern, assuming it makes herbal medicine untrustworthy. However, these factors don't prevent us from applying receptor theory. They simply indicate that the effects of an herbal medicine may vary somewhat between batches. And while the reality of variability in herbal medicines may seem messy to today's model of pharmacology, nature's inherent variability has not stopped herbal medicines from being used effectively for generations. So while there is variability in the composition of herbal medicines, that variability does not stop the practitioner from being practically useful.

Part of this is attributable to the fact that if one constituent is lower in a soup of actives, another helpful component might be higher. Generally speaking, herbal medicines are helpful not because they contain just one active ingredient but because the mix of their actives, often combined with the variable conglomeration of actives from multiple other plants, tend to help nudge a body system in the desirable direction. Herbalists typically lean toward a subtle adjustment in the desired direction, often achieved through a blend of ingredients that exhibit some variability while interacting with a range of different receptors, rather than a hammer blow that will instantly correct a perceived problem—the "magic bullet" approach. What's intriguing to consider is that both the intricate approach of herbal medicine, which embraces complexity, and the method of pharmaceuticals, which stresses consistency on all levels, assist the body in managing various stresses until it restores homeostasis.

Ultimately, if centuries and even millennia of experience indicate that despite the variability in herbal medicines, they can still achieve practical clinical effectiveness, this only suggests that the actions of herbal medicines are consistent with principles of modern drug-receptor theory and that herbal medicines do not need to be highly purified or isolated to be effective. Additionally, herbal medicine could be an opportunity to explore exciting new ways in which receptors respond within the context of intricate combinations of agonists and antagonists.

Complex and gentle herbal medicines are more consistent with the known complexity of the human body than the simpler, mechanistic "one disease, one target, one drug" model that has so influenced the foundation of conventional medicine. Indeed, the straightforward application of modern medicine is necessary and required frequently, but it beggars the imagination to conclude that every medical patient and situation requires *only* modern medicine or no medicine at all.

Abraham Maslow once suggested that a man with a hammer in his hand thinks everything is a nail.[95] Certainly, a profit-oriented drug company with a patented compound newly approved by FDA seems to think that drug is the best solution to a great many ills. By contrast, an herbal physician has a toolbox full of inexpensive, biodegradable, renewable, and time-tested ingredients that can be combined in countless ways to support individual health needs and goals. These medicines are safe and effective when their wise use is informed by accurate information, including experience.

Finally, as people differ in their responses to pharmaceutical drugs, they differ in their responses to herbal medicines too. Apart from allergic reactions to specific compounds, they are likely to respond less adversely to herbs used with wisdom than to conventional drugs, for many of the same reasons that also impact herbal efficacy. These include:

- Active ingredients in herbs are not isolated and concentrated, so the active ingredients (if known) tend to be used in smaller doses.

- Herbalists more often use herbs in combinations rather than using them individually, and these combinations typically require smaller doses than if using one of the same herbs in isolation.

- Herbal compounds often come in variant clusters, like gingerols or sanshools, where several related compounds may have similar and overlapping effects.

- Herbs have been used for many thousands of years, with vast populations, so those that are safe for most patients are well-known and those that are poisonous or have side effects also tend to be well-known; although, we do occasionally learn new things, even about herbs in common use.

Given the complexity of how receptors work and interact with their ligands, there is something to be said for the herbal approach, which is usually safe (when practiced with prudence) for most people and may generally move body function in the right direction by tickling many receptors, compared to single-ingredient drugs given with the intent of dominating and completely controlling the action of a single receptor that may not want to be told what to do for very long.

In summary, receptor theory gives a solid scientific foundation to both conventional and herbal medicine. However, very little about how receptor theory is applied clinically is simple, especially because of individual variations and adaptive responses during the course of drug use. Moreover, adverse effects can be difficult to identify and, again, vary from individual to individual while only fully manifesting after long-term use among many people. Oversimplification and lack of appreciation of these pitfalls lead to adverse outcomes. In many cases, while we understand mechanistically how some parts of herbal drugs work, we may have quite a bit more to learn about them because of their relative complexity and the equally complex environment (the human body) in which they operate. We will examine many of these issues in more detail as we proceed, beginning in the next chapter, where we enter the complex world of dose response relationships. How might these principles inform the development of more effective, personalized treatment strategies? This inquiry bridges our current understanding and ventures into the potential for tailored therapeutic approaches that accommodate individual physiological differences.

CHAPTER 4

Dose-Response Curves

Paracelsus, the father of toxicology, wrote in 1538, "What is there that is not poison? All things are poison and nothing is without poison. Only the dose determines that a thing is not a poison."[96]

Today, more than ever, we know this to be true. Powerful medicines can do good at the right doses for the right people, but *"first, do no harm"* remains one of the biggest challenges in medicine today.

Dose-response relationships are often positive—that is, if a small dose produces a small response, then a larger dose will produce a larger one, within limits. But even within an individual, the relationship is rarely linear: twice the dose doesn't produce twice the response. Powerful medicines often come with narrow safety margins, and although doctors can "titrate for effect," starting with a low dose and increasing until the desired effect is obtained, often neither patients nor their doctors are willing to spend that kind of time on any but the most difficult drug dosage problems. While drug doses are often adjusted for the weight of patients, many physicians (and patients) still find convenience in a simple, one-size-fits-all dosage solution—again, "take two tablets and call me in the morning."

Individuals differ in their responses to any drug, and in populations, the problem of variability becomes even larger and more complex. Individual responses vary with many factors, including age, sex, body mass and composition, genetics, epigenetics, microbiome, organ function and condition, and many more. While medical statistics can help us estimate the effect of a drug in a group of people, predicting individual therapeutic responses with precision is difficult. Moreover, drug approval studies are designed primarily to detect beneficial effects, while safety data is often less complete. This makes predicting adverse events in individuals even more difficult.

Dose-response curves help researchers and practitioners better understand the relationships between dose and response in individuals and populations. A dose-response (DR) curve is a graph that usually relates a dose (or blood concentration) on the horizontal (x) axis, with a response metric on the vertical (y) axis. Two or three different kinds of DR curves are commonly used in pharmacology: graded, quantal, and ordered.[97] Each has its purpose:

- Graded curves measure an analog response, such as the effect of caffeine on heart rate or blood pressure. Graded DR curves can be based on simple measures (e.g., body temperature or blood pressure) or calculated measures, such as a net change in blood pressure or percent of a maximal observed effect.

- A quantal response curve represents a response that is either present or absent, all or nothing. A quantal dose-response curve plots the presence of that quantal or binary response in a population, as the dosage increases. For example, quantal curves can show what percentage of a population experiences a specific drug effect at a given dose. Quantal response graphs were first used in toxicology to plot the lethal dose (LD) curve, which shows the percent of a population killed by increasing doses of a poison (and as Paracelsus said, everything is a poison). Researchers have adapted quantal response plots for various purposes, including various kinds of toxic dose (TD) curves and effective dose (ED) curves.

- Ordered curves simply plot multiple effects on the same chart. These could be different effects (e.g., ED, TD, and LD curves) for the same drug, or they can compare the relative effects of several different drugs. Ordered curves can be either graded or quantal, but quantal curves are more common, with many applications in pharmacology and toxicology.

Fitting Equations

In medicine, researchers use mathematical models and equations to interpret and explain data. Every mathematical model has its strengths, weaknesses, and limitations, but simpler models are generally easier to understand and often more helpful in practice than their more complex counterparts. In some cases, including too many parameters in a model can also decrease its accuracy when used.[98] Consistent with the scientific principle of parsimony, it's often best to use the simplest, adequate model that fits the data, even though the model is not perfect. In the words of the statistician G. E. P. Box, "All models are wrong but some are useful."[99] The complete picture is always layered: data, models, context, and experience in the field all play an important role in piecing together a solid understanding of dose-response patterns.

One of the simplest ways to model drug activity is by using the Hill equation to describe the relationship between drug concentration and drug effect.[100] Archibald Hill first used this equation in 1910 to describe oxygen binding to hemoglobin in blood. In general, one can express the Hill equation in various forms, typically incorporating up to four parameters:

- E_{min}: a lower or baseline limit, or minimal observed effect
- E_{max}: an upper limit, or maximal observed effect
- ED_{50}: the dose that produces a specific effect in 50% of the population
- n: the Hill coefficient, or exponent that determines the slope of the line at ED_{50}

However, a common variation of the Hill equation, especially in quantal data sets, fixes the lower bound at zero (the baseline at which there is no response, or 0%) and the upper bound at one (the maximal observed response is 100%). When fixing the upper and lower bounds in this way, we only need the last two parameters to define the curve. The International Union of Basic and Clinical Pharmacology (IUPHAR) gives the Hill equation for tissue response,[101] which, after a little simplification, becomes the equation below, which we used in the accompanying figures:

$$\%E_{max} = E\,/\,E_{max} = 1\,/\,(\,1 + (ED_{50}\,/\,D)^n\,)$$

This plots the percentage of maximal effect ($E\,/\,E_{max}$) as a function of dosage (D), where ED_{50} is the half-maximal effective dose and n is the Hill coefficient.

The Hill equation can also describe drug agonist activity at a receptor. In that case, the Hill coefficient describes binding cooperativity, where n = 1 is independence, n < 1 indicates negative cooperation (interference), and n > 1 indicates positive cooperation. Hemoglobin, for example, can bind up to four oxygen molecules and has a Hill coefficient between 2.7 and 3, depending on the physiological properties of the solution.[102] It is significantly easier for a hemoglobin molecule to bind another oxygen atom when it has already done so.

While the Hill equation is the most common way to model drug activity, we should recognize the assumptions in this approach. Sometimes, the equation may not nicely fit the data observed. For example, sometimes a drug may have both inhibitory and stimulatory effects at different doses. Other times, unlike in the figures below, the dose-response pattern has two inflection points. In such situations, a standard Hill curve won't fit the data well.[103] When it fits the data, the Hill equation tells us a lot about the near-linear responses observed near the mean, where the therapeutic window generally lies and it may also explain diminishing responses, which we usually observe at the upper end of the curve. However, we often have much less information about the lower end of the curve, where any response signal may blend with background noise. Signal to noise ratio (SNR[104]), a common concept in many engineering fields, may need to be more closely examined in the pharmacological setting, especially if the lower end of the curve carries sparse but important drug safety signals.

Graded Dose-Response Curves

Figure 3-1 gives a simple example of graded Hill dose-response curves for several fictional drugs:

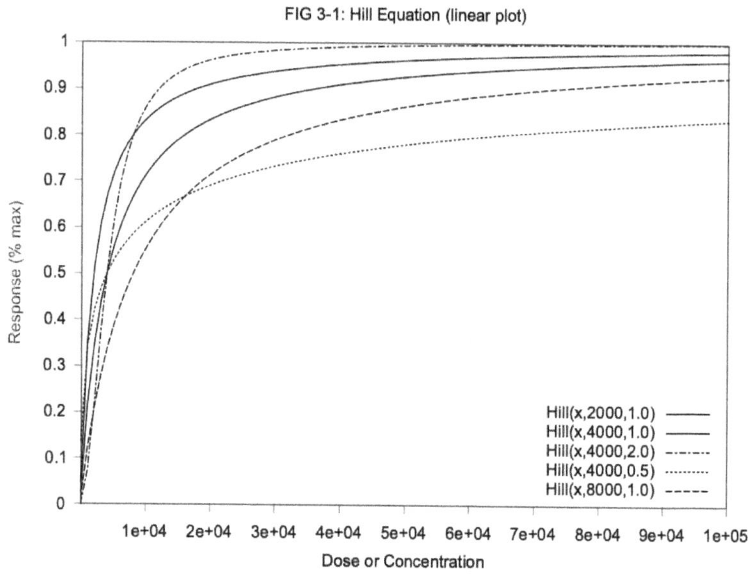

In most cases, E_{min} is zero, meaning that when there is no dose, there is no effect, but in some cases, E_{min} can be a baseline physiological measure and E_{max} the highest possible or desirable level. Some researchers also discuss a "threshold dose" below which a drug has no significant effect, but the ED_{50} and slope are probably the most important elements in interpreting the curve for clinical purposes.

The example shows three effective doses (ED_{50}) at 2,000, 4,000, and 8,000 dosage units, with three different slopes at the 4,000 dosage level. When the slopes are equal, a drug with a lower ED_{50} is more potent, with a greater effect at any given dose along the curve. Similarly, if the ED_{50} is the same for two drugs, the one with a steeper slope is more potent, reaching higher effects more quickly.

These principles explain why for the sake of efficacy, drugs with lower ED_{50} and steeper slopes would be preferred—they're more potent.

However, aspects of safety, such as adverse effects and how a drug interacts with other medications, also play crucial roles in determining the best treatment option. Potency isn't the whole picture.

Semilog Curves

Dosages of different drugs and other substances can vary widely. Air, food, and water intake are all measured in kilograms per day (1e3), whereas the dosing for trace minerals is typically in micrograms (1e-6). As a result, it often helps to put dosages on a logarithmic scale to make comparisons easier. This approach can also help us place information about the most commonly used doses in the more linear portions of the dose-response curve in the center of the figure.

Figure 3-2 plots exactly the same data as figure 3-1, but uses a semilog scale (logarithmic on x-axis only). This produces a series of sigmoid (s-shaped) curves that are more common in medical and especially pharmacological contexts:

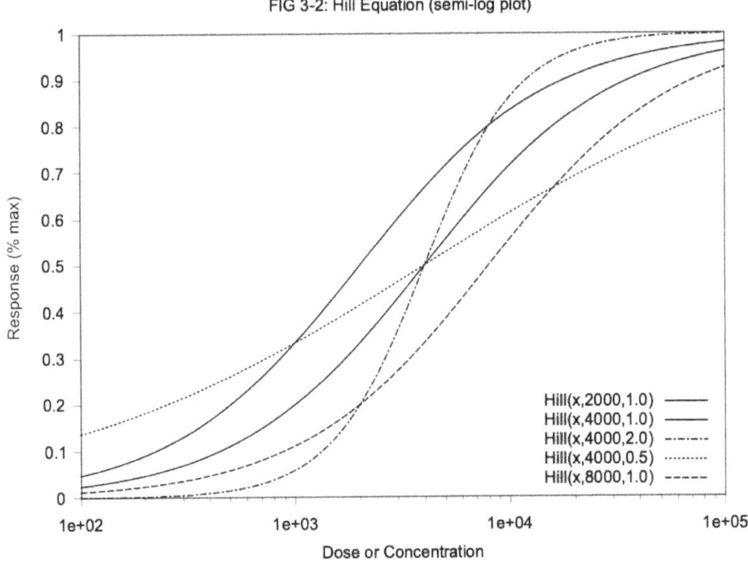

Semilog plots, with their distinctive sigmoid curves, are so common in medicine that some medical professionals may find alternative formats to present dose-response information uncomfortable. However, while a semilog plot affects the way the curve appears on a graph, it has no effect on the underlying model or the collected data. The dose-response data relationships remain exactly the same, whether plotted on a linear or logarithmic scale.

Quantal Curves

Individuals vary in their responses to drugs, just as they vary in height, weight, strength, lung capacity, and other characteristics. Individual variations around the mean generally form the bell-shaped curve of a statistical standard distribution (fig. 3-3). Whether we're talking about alcohol, caffeine, or any other drug, we all know people who respond differently than most. Graded response curves can show how dose is associated with response in a population. However, quantal response curves are better for tracking what percentage of a population has responded at any given dose, which, along with the information from a graded response curve, helps when making decisions for individual patients.

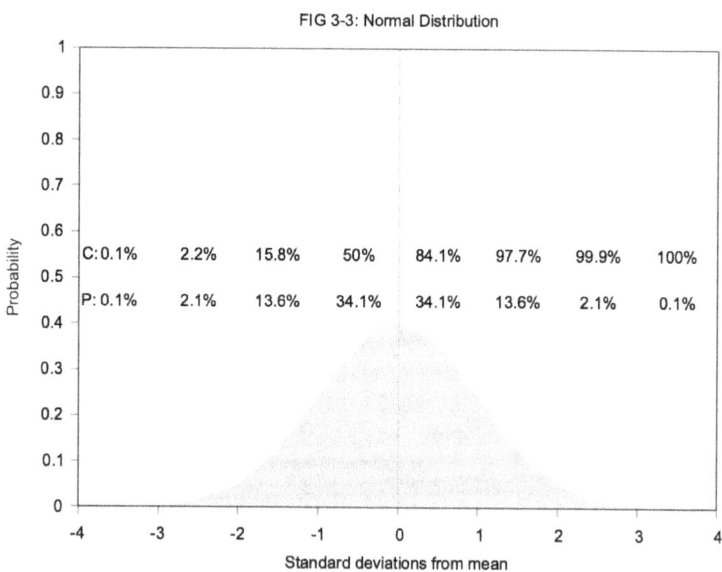

In standard distributions, mean (mu) and standard deviation (sigma) differ across populations. An individual's response can range from highly responsive (experiencing effects at lower dosages) to relatively unresponsive. However, the probability values (p-values) for each standard deviation interval in a bell curve, like the one in figure 3-3, remain constant: 34.1%, 13.6%, 2.1%, and 0.1% for each successive standard deviation from the mean. The row marked "P" displays these p-values for each interval, while the cumulative values (one-tailed z-values), labeled "C," show the total percentage affected up to and including each interval, moving from left to right. As the dosage increases, we observe additional effects, and the cumulative percentage of affected individuals rises toward 100%. It's important to remember that the most reliable data typically lie near the center, while the edges are less well known and, indeed, less knowable—like scorpions, statistics carry their sting in the long tails of the bell curve.

Quantal measures help us determine where various portions of the population fall on this bell curve. Quantal refers to an all-or-none (binary) physiological response, like dead or alive, and the first quantal response curves were probably LD curves used in toxicology. Another quantal measure is the inebriometer used to measure the effect of inhaled anesthetics on fruit flies: it counts the flies as they progressively lose the ability to fly or crawl and fall to the device's bottom. Death, REM sleep, unconsciousness, spasm, and fibrillation are examples of naturally quantal responses—they represent a fairly sudden change in a binary state.

With a carefully defined binary test, we can convert almost any graded response to a quantal count. Did the patient have another heart attack within a year? Did the drug reduce perceived pain by at least 20%? On the other hand, a poorly defined quantal question can be tough to measure. When do symptoms disappear completely? When does a fever begin? Even for death, the simplest quantal case, it matters whether the observation occurs minutes or weeks after dosage. It's generally more efficient to choose a simple, easily measured quantal threshold, like a reduction in fever of one degree centigrade, than to discern a signal that is difficult to separate from background noise, such as exact onset or complete end of fever or other symptoms.

Tracking a quantal response across varying doses reveals the variation in response seen in individuals and groups of individuals who respond at a particular dose. This approach involves plotting these responses in a histogram, as figure 3-4 illustrates. For this example, we cribbed our fifty-six undefined data points from the quantal dose-response page of Alex Yarsev's excellent Deranged Physiology website.[105] At each incremental dosage level, researchers count the new quantal responses and place them into the successive intervals of a histogram (fig. 3-4). In this example, they form a standard probability bell curve, showing the frequency of response at different dosages.

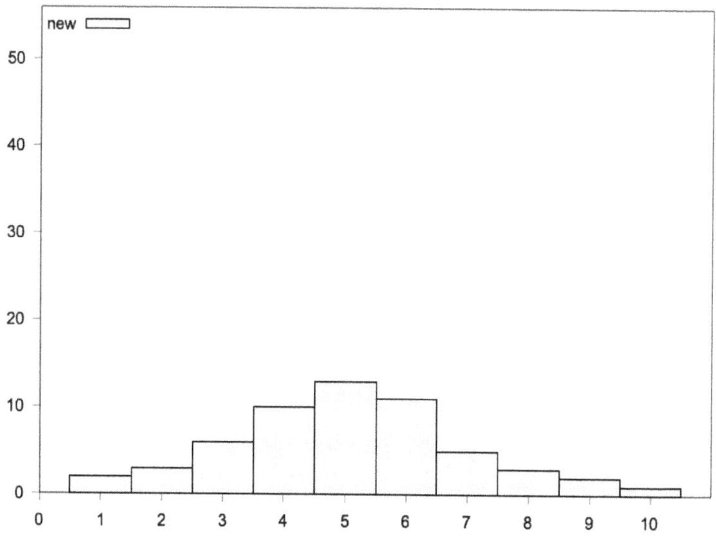

FIG 3-4: Simple quantal histogram (n=56)

As the quantal responses accumulate with increasing doses, each bin builds on the sum of the prior (lower-dose) bins, creating a stepped histogram, shown in figure 3-5. These data points undergo a smoothing process to shape into a sigmoid cumulative probability curve, also presented in figure 3-5.

FIG 3-5: Stepped quantal histogram (with sigmoid curve, n=56)

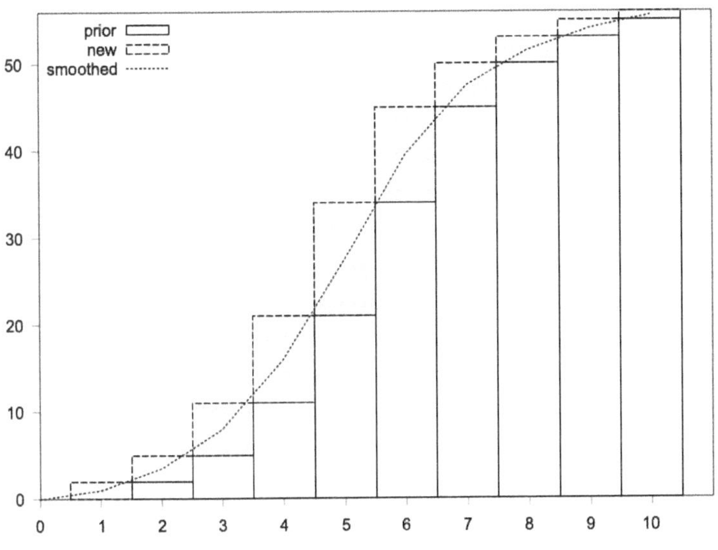

There are several important points to remember about the cumulative quantal curve:

- The quantal test determines the location of the curve midpoint (ED_{50}). If we change the test (e.g., observation time for death, or the clinical definition of "effective"), the ED_{50} will shift accordingly.
- The variability of the quantal response determines the slope of the curve. Small variances will produce steep curves, while broad variances will produce shallow ones.
- From a clinical perspective, the most important data typically fall near the midpoint of the dose-response curve. The ED_{50} is a key reference for understanding drug efficacy. We have much less data about individuals who fall more than one to two SD either above or below the mean, or ED_{50}.

Finally, we should remember that the lethal dose quantal curve is natural, intuitive, and valuable. If the quantal primary or desired drug effect is carefully defined, an ED curve also makes a lot of sense. But the often-assumed TD curve between the ED and LD curves is a different kettle of fish, as we will examine in more detail below. Too often, we assume a single TD curve that falls somewhere between the ED and LD curves. But in reality, there may be separate curves for every side effect, adverse event, or form of toxicity we could imagine. As with all quantal curves, the devil is in the definitions.

Ordered Response Curves

Researchers often use ordered quantal curves to demonstrate the varied effects of a single drug. For example, general anesthetics often provide different effects at successively higher doses: sedation, drowsiness, agitation, stupor, sleep, unconsciousness, anesthesia, central nervous system depression, and (eventually) death. Doctors need to know where the patient is on each of these curves to maintain proper anesthesia for surgery. Patients may be high or low on the sensitivity scale for various steps, making them unsuitable candidates for a particular drug, and this may only become apparent once the procedure has begun.

Researchers often use an ordered set of quantal response curves (including ED, TD, and LD) to examine various drugs' relative safety and efficacy. For example, when comparing drugs, a drug that gets more quantal response at a lower dose level (lower ED_{50}) is more potent, while a drug with a steeper quantal ED slope effectively treats a wide range of individuals within a narrower dosage range, possibly giving it a narrower therapeutic window. Neither measure considered alone is adequate. All else being equal (which is never the case), a less potent drug whose change in effect (whether graded or quantal) can be managed with gradual dose changes may be a better choice in clinical practice.

Therapeutic Index

One of the most important safety measures for drugs is the therapeutic index (TI), a measure of the safety margin between the doses usually prescribed or used in practice and the dose that would be toxic or lethal. In animal studies, the formula is usually given as LD_{50}/ED_{50}, whereas in human medicine it takes the more conservative form of TD_{50}/ED_{50}. Either way, the idea is that a medicine whose ED_{50} is much lower than its LD_{50} or TD_{50} is safer than a drug whose ED_{50} is dangerously close to its TD_{50} or LD_{50}.

In practice, the TI of many drugs can be large, and safe use is likely. Remifentanil, a fast-acting opioid painkiller used intravenously for short-term effect around surgery, is reputed to have a TI of about 33,000.[106] On the other hand, drugs such as warfarin and digoxin have a TI of roughly 2,[107] and doctors must monitor them very closely to prevent catastrophic consequences. Other drugs fall between these extremes; the commonly used drug Prozac has a TI of 100.[108]

However, a TI of 100 or more, while appearing safe, doesn't guarantee safety if a drug is prescribed at levels many times higher than the ED_{50}, and problems can occur with long-term use that don't appear with a single use. For example, one correct dose of an opiate may be quite safe, but the risk of abuse disorders goes up with longer-term use and higher doses. Thus, it may make sense to consider an "effective TI" (our term) incorporating real-world information about dosage and toxicity in conditions closer to common use. For example, if physicians commonly prescribe a drug at a dose representing an ED_{60} or ED_{75}, they could divide the TD_{50} by that dose, instead of the ED_{50}, which is not commonly used.

Pairing the usual or effective TI with adverse event data enhances its clinical usefulness. Consider, for example, a drug that has an acute TD_{50} of 100 mg and an ED_{50} of 10 mg but is actually commonly prescribed around the ED_{75} level, a dose that turns out to be 20 mg. Moreover, most patients use the drug over many years. Finally, we know from clinical data that with use of the drug for over a year, there is a 1% chance of hepatotoxicity. Then instead of reporting a TI of 10, derived by simply dividing the TD_{50} of 100 mg by the seldom-used ED_{50} of 10 mg, we could derive and report an effective TI by dividing the TD_{50} by the ED_{75} that is actually used and report the information as "Effective TI of 5, 1% risk of hepatotoxicity with use over one year."

Some common drugs and substances are surprisingly dangerous: acetaminophen (Tylenol) has a TI of about 10,[109] and even water can be toxic if consumed at roughly four to six times normal rates. Fortunately, drinking too much water is physically painful, so toxicity doesn't happen often. Cocaine and alcohol have TIs of about 15 and 10,[110] respectively, but because abuse causes tolerance, and overdose is relatively painless, serious adverse events are common.

Other safety measures exist, including the margin of safety (MOS). One calculates this by dividing the toxic dose for 1% of the population (TD_{01}) by the effective dose for 99% of the population (ED_{99}). Different drugs may have different shapes of ED and TD curves, which makes for wide variability in MOS calculations.[111]

Many common herbal medicines would seem to have a forgiving TI or are otherwise difficult to overdose due to taste, bulk, or other factors. The rate of serious adverse events reported for dietary supplements (which includes herbal medicines) is a small fraction of the rate for prescription drugs,[112,113] even though 35% of the US population takes herbal supplements.[114]

Climbing the Curve: Dosages above ED_{50}

One of the biggest issues with dosing pharmaceutical drugs is that the ED_{50} only gets the desired response for half the population. Prescribers want drugs that work for most or nearly all of their patients, not just half of them. As a result, many may consider the ED_{50} as the minimum acceptable practical dosage. In the conventional "one disease, one target, one drug" medical model, there's typically just one ED curve for a given drug and intended use.

To increase the drug's effect for a larger portion of the population, the dosage often moves up the curve from the ED_{50}, toward the ED_{70}, ED_{90}, or even ED_{95}. However, these more effective levels can require much larger doses. Consequently, doctors commonly prescribe many drugs at dosages ten, twenty, or even fifty times higher than the ED_{50} dose. Statin drugs, for example, are often prescribed at forty times their ED_{50}.[115] Other examples of drugs that may commonly be prescribed at doses many times their ED_{50} include the heart failure drug candesartan and many antidepressant SSRIs.[116] Prescribing drugs at levels well beyond their ED_{50} leads inevitably to an increase in adverse events.

So long as we follow the "one disease, one target, one drug" model, we find ourselves on the horns of a dilemma: the only way to get more therapeutic effect from a single drug is a higher effective dose (ED), which pushes us further up the toxicity curves (TD/LD) as well.

Our first set of graded response curves (figs. 3-1 and 3-2, above) intentionally showed half-maximal response rates that were fairly close together (multiples of 3x) to effectively demonstrate the difference between linear and logarithmic scales on the same data set. In practice, most dose-response graphs are semilogarithmic to cover wider variations in dosage, so examining a more typical (or conservative) set of curves may be helpful.

In this example (fig. 3-6), we have intentionally selected curves at 100x intervals to represent a drug that would usually be considered relatively safe. This diagram shows three curves: ED, TD, and LD, from left to right. Because the LD_{50} is 10,000 times higher than the ED_{50} this drug has a TI of 10,000:1 when using the LD_{50} in the calculation and a TI of 100:1 when TD_{50} (marked "TI" on the figure) is used to calculate the ratio. Again, in practice the LD_{50} is commonly used in animal studies, while the TD_{50} is preferred for human populations.

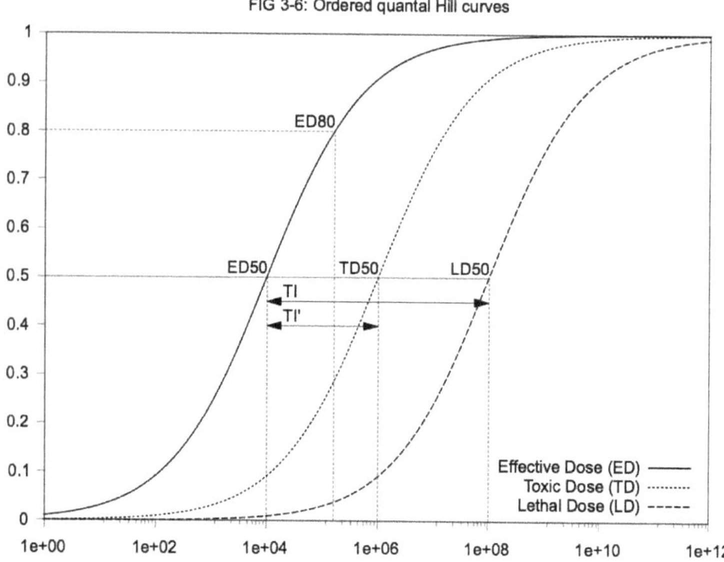

For the sake of demonstration, in this figure, we selected a uniform Hill slope of 0.5 for all three curves to clearly demonstrate that the top of one curve can significantly overlap the bottom of the next, even when the curves are relatively widely spaced. At the ED_{50} for this fictional drug, if we follow that dosage level down to the other two curves, we note that toxicity on the TD curve is already nearing 10%, and lethality (LD) is nonzero. If we push up the ED curve to the ED_{80}, toxicity is nearing 30%, while lethality is almost 4%. This increase from ED_{50} to ED_{80} yields a 60% improvement in drug efficacy. However, it also leads to a substantial rise in adverse effects: a roughly 200% increase in toxicity and a 300% surge in fatalities—no bargain by anyone's standards. So a "safe" TI (no matter which formula we pick) is no safety guarantee. Unless we have a clear idea how the various curves are positioned and interact with each other, we can easily get ourselves into trouble.

Still, there may be individual patients who would absolutely benefit from this drug. It might even save their lives. But we'd need to be very careful in selecting this drug, perhaps starting much lower (say, ED_{10}), titrating carefully for effect while monitoring closely for toxicity, and carefully assessing the risks and benefits for each case.

One of the problems with the TD curve is that there isn't actually just one—there are in fact many possible TDs. Toxicity can be acute, chronic, or subchronic; cumulative or not; temporary, permanent, or reversible. There may be interactions with other drugs that lead to toxicity or cellular congestion of drugs due to competition for excretory channels. There might also be toxicities due to allergic reactions, genetic mutations, or other factors. Textbooks sometimes discuss mild, nuisance, and acute toxicity curves, but even these demarcations probably don't capture the real complexity of the toxicity landscape or ensure that all toxicity curves are completely defined. So to think of a single TD curve, let alone a single TD_{50}, may be a gross oversimplification. In this context, the lethality LD_{50} may be more reliable, even though it may be derived from animal (we hope) studies, which may differ from human effects.

Similarly, many drugs can be used for a variety of different primary effects, each with its own unique ED curve. The complexity of the relationships between these various ED, TD, and LD curves can quickly become overwhelming. But if it's any consolation, there is only one LD curve, and we truly hope we never accidentally find it.

Individual Variations

It isn't uncommon for people to describe themselves as relatively sensitive or insensitive to drugs in general or to a specific drug. Certainly, we know that a sickly great-grandmother and an Olympic weight lifter in training won't respond identically to most drugs, but even similar people respond differently. They may be hypersensitive to one drug, relatively resistant to another, and more or less average in response to others. Some people may get jittery with caffeine from one cup of coffee while others drink several cups a day without much effect on mood. Some people feel alert when taking a single dose of diphenhydramine, and others go to sleep. Individuals have quirks concerning any single drug's various ED, TD, or LD curves: they may be high on one, low on another, and average for others.

Before we move on, let's consider another example in which we commonly analyze multiple ordered dose-response curves together. Surgery often requires general anesthetics, which may have several successive effects at increasing dosages, such as (in order from left to right) drowsiness, nausea, unconsciousness, respiratory depression, and death. In this situation, an anesthesiologist has a specific goal: to induce unconsciousness but not respiratory depression or death. Since nausea, and especially vomiting, may interfere with surgery and recovery, the object is to pass through the nausea curve as quickly as possible.

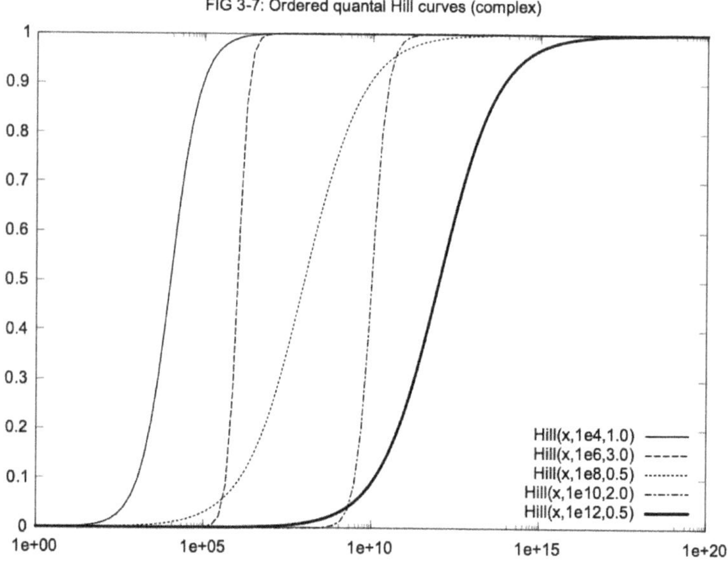

FIG 3-7: Ordered quantal Hill curves (complex)

Remember that in quantal curves, the Hill coefficient (slope) measures the variability of the dose-response relationship in different individuals that make up a population. Some drugs (or effects) will have wider ranges of variability than others, producing shallower slopes and a wider radius to the curves. There is no reason to assume the slope is 1 or any other number on a quantal curve. Similarly, the spacing between curves may differ widely, changing the possible points of overlap. In practice, Hill coefficients for quantal curves are seldom reported and often very hard to find.

Please note that we have assumed that we can determine and plot the position and slope of these illustrative curves based on the presence of some imaginary but available data. Researchers base LD curves on animal models in practice and rarely know them in much detail for humans. Toxicity curves are similarly difficult to obtain with ethical experimentation. Safety data are often obtained during clinical efficacy trials, without the studies being constructed or powered to focus on toxic events. Thus, the toxicity curves of a drug are not often fully appreciated and defined before drug approval, as evidenced by the fact that about a quarter of drugs need the addition of significant safety warnings or to be removed from market after they are made available to patients.[117]

Both before and after drug approval, new drug safety information comes primarily from adverse event reports. These data do not align with the half-maximal portion of these curves where we could calculate a mean and standard deviation. Instead, this is usually sparse, infrequent data, collected (hopefully) at the lower end of the population curve's tail and mixed with unrelated background noise, such as random heart attacks or other toxicological events unrelated to the study. Trying to estimate the shape and location of these curves from the limited data available is a bit like trying to estimate the weight of an elephant by the size and shape of the tip of its tail. In fact, it might be worse, because with background noise, you're never even sure if the tail you're looking at belongs to the right elephant!

TD and LD curves are important, even if they aren't fully and clearly defined. Indeed, the LD curve is about as consequential as it gets. The challenge of pharmacovigilance is very real—tests on a small population of animals or people may not translate well into real-world safety experience with a larger population and over a much longer period of time.

Small wonder that many approved drugs are eventually withdrawn from the market due to safety concerns.

We should also mention in passing that efficacy testing standards tend to increase the safety concerns with any drug. Proving efficacy with statistical rigor requires a high signal-to-noise ratio, which encourages higher dosing during investigation. Higher dosing often gets approval but also increases risk of harm. In statistical efficacy testing, the biggest hammer always wins, but is the biggest hammer always the best option? Moreover, medical treatment raises a fundamental question: are we treating populations with statistical effects, or do we focus on individuals needing tailored options based on their unique response and tolerance? *We can't deliver the best clinical solution to individual patients if we treat them based solely on population data.*

Now that we have delved deep into the world of dose-response curves and we understand the usefulness of these tools as well as some of their limitations, it is helpful to stand back a little and ask an important question: can the long-standing empirical data obtained through centuries of use of herbal remedies provide a more direct and accessible understanding of their safety and efficacy than the relatively controlled data used to construct the dose-response curves of modern pharmacology? We believe it may. For example, while recent clinical trial evidence is opening up minds in the West to the usefulness of Tongxinluo, a medicine made in China from traditional herbal and insect ingredients to prevent heart attacks,[118] practitioners in China informed the creation of this combination of ingredients based on knowledge gained through many centuries of ingredient use. Experience counts.

What's Different with Herbal Medicine?

Many ancient herbal traditions, including traditional Chinese and Ayurvedic medicine, have long abandoned (or never used) the simplistic "one disease, one target, one drug" model that Western medicine often still uses. Where modern medicine is just now moving from a disease model to a patient-centered approach,[119] herbal medicine has always been holistic and patient-centered.

Herbal medicine is more complex than conventional pharmaceuticals, as we have introduced above. While most conventional drugs are composed of a single chemical compound, herbal medicines may have hundreds of compounds, active and inactive (and often unknown). They may vary in potency by region, altitude, soil and weather conditions, grower, and season. They may be dried or processed differently. In short, they are every bit as variable as the individuals that use them. How, then, can they offer any advantage over the known effects of a single drug?

As we have seen, the biggest variable in the pharmaceutical equation is how a unique individual responds to a drug. Individuals also respond differently to herbs, but since herbs are typically not as concentrated as drugs, the variations aren't as dramatic.

In herbal medical practice, two important approaches are highly encouraged:

1) Conservative practice using gentle herbs and combinations that are well-known and used for many years and

2) Early intervention to prevent or correct problems before they become serious.

When herbalists do innovate, they often build on patterns recognized for many years. Rather than move up the ED curve with a single powerful ingredient, they will likely move down the curve, combining several ingredients with similar or complementary effects. Individuals who do not respond to one ingredient may find that they respond to others, while those who might experience negative effects from a particular ingredient are likely to experience milder effects when that ingredient is used in combination with others at a relatively small dose. Intelligent formula design using small amounts of ingredients in combination can also reduce known or likely side effects of single ingredients. And combining herbs allows multiple mechanisms to work together to support a body system or function, such as the anti-nausea effects of ginger combined with the antispasmodic effects of peppermint. Many herbal remedies have a tonic nature, which means that instead of overpowering a body system, they help the body maintain or restore its self-regulating capabilities. These kinds of approaches are only now finding their way into conventional medicine but have been part of the herbal tradition for many centuries.

Just as conventional medicine has done for the past century, herbalists could choose to isolate, concentrate, and administer herbal compounds in a similar manner. To the extent that herbal medicine goes down that path, it can expect the same results as these dose-response curves suggest—trading ever-increasing potency and dosage for increased efficacy, but always at a greater risk of adverse events.

Herbal medicine, while not replacing modern medicine, presents a sensible alternative with unique benefits, particularly for preventing or addressing early-stage health issues. The benefits of a traditional herbal approach, which emphasizes combinations of low doses of multiple ingredients, provide less opportunity to travel upward on a dose-response curve and trade safety for efficacy.

CHAPTER 5

Low Dose Therapy as the Common Conclusion of Multiple Dose-Response Models

Different Kinds of Pharmacological Curves

In the last chapter, we explored a typical sigmoidal dose-response curve that allows for the estimation of an effective dose 50 (ED_{50}) in a population, commonly used as a model of drug dose-response in today's view of pharmacology. Ascension up such a curve increases the probability of toxicity as the advancement in efficacy slows. In this chapter, we explore a different dimension of dose-response, the biphasic or hormetic response, and suggest that given the understanding this model provides, low-dose therapy again asserts itself as a preferable approach to formulation.

In hormetic dose-response, an intervention has a stimulatory effect at a low dose but an inhibitory effect at a higher dose. For example, low doses of ethanol in rats stimulate social behavior while larger doses inhibit it. Below is a figure illustrating a hypothetical example of an agent that stimulates cell growth at lower concentrations but inhibits growth at higher concentrations.

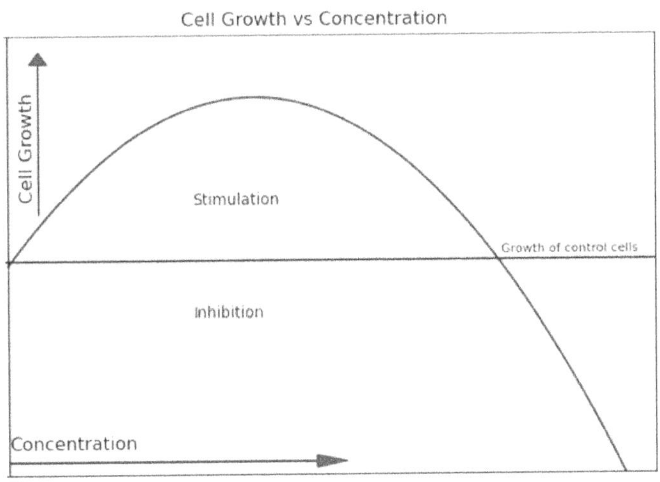

History of the Scientific Community's Relationship with Hormetic Dose Response

Calabrese has published an excellent review on the scientific community's complex relationship with the hormetic dose response.[120] Hugo Schulz, a contemporary of Louis Pasteur and Robert Koch, first described this dose-response pattern. He did his microbiological research at Greifswald University in Germany and began publishing his findings in the 1880s. Working with disinfectants that killed yeast (inhibited fermentation) at high doses, he noted that there was an "indifference point" below which he repeatedly observed stimulatory effects. He describes his work in this way:[121]

Sometimes, when working with substances that needed to be examined for their effectiveness in comparison to the inducers of yeast fermentation, initially working together with my assistant, Gottfried Hoffmann, I found in formic acid and also in other substances the marvelous occurrence that if I got below their indifference point, i.e., if, for example, I worked with less formic acid than was required to halt the appearance of its anti-fermentative property, that all at once the carbon dioxide production became distinctly higher than in the controls processed without the formic acid addition. I first thought, as is obvious, that there had been some kind of experimental or observation error. But the appearance of the overproduction continually repeated itself under the same conditions. First I did not know how to deal with it, and in any event at that time still did not realize that I had experimentally proved the first theorem of Arndt's fundamental law of biology.

Schulz and his colleague, Rudolf Arndt, later claimed that their observations of a hormetic response pattern explained the effectiveness of homeopathy, provided that one does not dilute the substances in the remedies beyond Avogadro's number. Because of this, Schulz and Arndt were highly criticized by the proponents of other dose-response models and their work was largely rejected.[122] This was a tragedy, mainly because their research was later corroborated[123] and the principle of a biphasic response was reported in other biological models.[124,125] Eventually, however, as examples of hormetic response continued to accumulate—and owing much to Calabrese's team of researchers—the hormetic dose response became recognized as a generalizable principle of the biological sciences,[126] incorporating the concepts of additivity and synergy.[127]

The hormetic response can be illustrated with resveratrol. At low concentrations (0.625 and 1.25 mcg/ml), resveratrol has a stimulatory effect on gamma-interferon and interleukin-2 production of peripheral blood mononuclear cells (PBMCs), while doses above this amount inhibit secretion of these cytokines. Likewise, multiple levels of resveratrol below 2.5 mcg/ml consistently increase interleukin-4 production, while concentrations above this amount are increasingly inhibitory. Reports also show a hormetic response regarding resveratrol's effects on PBMC viability and replication; low concentrations of resveratrol stimulate, while larger concentrations inhibit.[128]

A further example of a hormetic response is the varying effect of different concentrations of saponins from the well-known adaptogenic herb *Panax notoginseng* on cell proliferation.[129] Lower concentrations of saponins increase the proliferation of PC12 cells, with a peak increase of 30.3% at 0.12 mg/ml. This effect gradually declines with increasing doses until 4 mg/ml produces an inhibitory effect.

It is important to remember that not every hormetic response may be desirable. For instance, berberine has been shown in vitro to have stimulatory effects on cancer cell lines at concentrations between 1.25 and 5 μM and inhibitory effects at higher concentrations between 10 and 80 µM.[130] This highlights the need for a better understanding of the effects of low-dose therapies in vivo, including the cumulative effects of low-dose combination therapies.

While great insight into this issue will come from the combination of basic science research and longer-term clinical trials, we would argue that there is also value in learning from empirical formulation methods used for centuries. For example, in traditional Chinese medicine (TCM), creating an herbal formula isn't just about mixing a main, or "monarch," herb with a "minister" herb that boosts its effects. It's also important to include an "assistant" herb. Practitioners of TCM specifically add this assistant herb to counteract any toxicity from the monarch and minister herbs.[131] Learnings accumulated over centuries with this approach may tend to lead to a sum of hormetic responses that is generally beneficial.

At this point, it may be helpful to consider several questions: if many herbs combined in low doses present the body with multiple opportunities for hormetic responses and low-potency homeopathics (still containing low amounts of chemicals from source materials) also induce hormetic responses, is the line drawn between the two therapeutic categories an artificial one? If both approaches are different means of achieving a favorable balance of hormetic responses, could we not group them under a larger umbrella of hormetic-response inducers? Lastly, if the therapeutic advantage of low-dose combination therapy comes from the cumulative effects of hormetic responses, can healing occur in many situations without any single ingredient reaching an ED_{50} on a standard dose-response curve? The effects of hormetic responses seem a very plausible avenue for explaining the long-observed benefits of TCM[132] and the formulas of other healing systems, such as Ayurveda, that commonly mix many whole herbal and other medicinal ingredients together in low amounts. Indeed, a hormetic dose response is of particular interest to naturopathic physicians and may even be seen as a unifying dose-response model across multiple naturopathic modalities.

Based on a collective view of the information above and that presented in our review of the typical dose-response model, one intriguing observation is that both descriptions of dose-response provide reasons to pursue low-dose combination therapy in practice. In the case of hormetic dose-responses, seeking to capture beneficial stimulatory effects of low amounts of multiple ingredients makes sense. In the case of a sigmoidal dose-response, combining low doses of medicines helps avoid unacceptable trade-offs between efficacy and safety as the dose of a single drug increases. Thus, whether one feels more intellectual affinity for a typical, sigmoidal dose-response curve or finds joy and utility in seeking to become a respectable hormetic response specialist, both dose-response models suggest low-dose combination therapy as a logical path forward.

At this point, you probably have a greater appreciation for how medicines act in the body and the various kinds of dose-response relationships. Still, there are many individual factors that affect how a medicine, either herbal formulation or prescription drug, ultimately impacts a given individual. To use medicines with the greatest possible safety and efficacy, we must consider individual factors, as we discuss in the following chapter.

CHAPTER 6

Individual Variation in Drug Response

While studies can help us understand overall patterns of drug effects in larger populations, many factors affect an individual's clinical response. In this chapter, we explore examples of how disease, aging, gender, and genetic variation play important roles in shaping individual responses to drug therapy.

Effects of Disease on Pharmacokinetics and Pharmacodynamics

Probably the most obvious diseases that impact a person's sensitivity to drugs are diseases of the liver. While other organs, such as the gut and kidneys, are also important in drug metabolism, the liver serves as a main site of drug metabolism, and changes in its functional tissue can alter drug pharmacokinetics. However, insults to liver tissue may be acute or chronic; mediated by different causes such as viruses, the effects of poisoning, or autoimmunity; and occur in varying degrees of severity.[133] Thus the exact impact of liver disease on drug metabolism will vary from one person to another. Talal provides a helpful review of noninvasive imaging and functional tests that may be most useful in assessing the liver's potential to impact drug pharmacokinetics.[134]

In naturopathic medical school, an introductory lecture frequently emphasizes the role of inflammation as a common and crucial intermediary between health and different states of disease. It turns out that the common facilitator of disease, inflammation, also has a rather complex relationship with drug pharmacokinetics and pharmacodynamics. It is not uncommon, for example, for patients with cirrhosis to show elevated markers of inflammation, including TNF alpha and IL-6, which may be elevated in response to bacterial translocation from the gut to the liver.[135] Elevations of IL-6 may be particularly significant as the inflammatory response marked with its increase is known to suppress hepatocyte CYP activity.[136] This suppression can affect pharmacokinetics by increasing drug concentration. In an interesting example of how the management of systemic disease can impact drug metabolism, suppression of CYP3A, CYP2C9, and CYP2C19 activity in patients with rheumatoid arthritis (RA) is known to be reversed by administration of a monoclonal antibody to soluble interleukin-6 (IL-6).[137] A similar finding of reversing CYP3A4 suppression in patients with RA is shown with a monoclonal antibody to IL-6 receptor.[138]

However, inflammation-driven changes in pharmacokinetics do not always translate into predictable changes in pharmacodynamics. For instance, in one study, while patients with RA showed significantly higher serum levels of the drug verapamil in association with increasing levels of IL-6, the ability of the drug to actually prolong the PR-interval decreased and the effect of the drug on heart rate and blood pressure did not increase. This pattern of changes may be due to receptor down-regulation.[139] A similar pattern is seen in patients with the inflammation of active Crohn's disease.[140] In patients with active disease, the concentration of verapamil increases, but this does not coincide with an enhanced pharmacodynamic effect of verapamil; conversely, reducing the severity of the inflammatory disease increases drug response despite lower drug concentration. These findings may be early evidence of a generalized principle: that dealing with inflammation must be a priority in order to ensure predictable pharmacodynamics.

Effects of Aging

The pharmacokinetics and pharmacodynamics of many drugs become less tightly regulated as we age. Many factors, such as changes in organ weight and the level of drug receptors, may contribute to these changes.

However, decreases in hepatic and renal blood flow in the older population seem to be among the most important causes of reduced drug clearance (the volume of plasma cleared of a drug in a specific time) and steady increases in area under the curve (AUC) of many drugs after the age of seventy.[141] The sensitivity merited in prescribing to the geriatric population underpins the axiom "start low and go slow."[142] An example is metabolism of O-desmethyltramadol (ODM), the active metabolite of tramadol. In comparing an aging group with mild renal insufficiency (common in a geriatric population) and a younger group, researchers found that the older group took significantly longer to reach maximal plasma concentrations of ODM and that the subsequent decline in ODM concentration also took significantly longer. There was also a 15% higher maximum possible treatment effect in the older group, suggesting both an opportunity for increased benefit and a greater potential for adverse effects in the elderly.[143] Other examples of drugs, among many, that demonstrate a tendency for decreased clearance and increased concentration in older patients prone to decreasing hepatic and renal function are cefoperazone[144] and clarithromycin.[145]

Unfortunately, with identified differences in pharmacokinetics, it is not always clear whether these changes equate to clinically meaningful changes in pharmacodynamics or safety outcomes. For example, while in an elderly population, there is a relatively large decrease in clearance of lisinopril,[146] this does not seem to substantially impact its clinical effects.[147] Carefully clarifying meaningful pharmacodynamic differences between older and younger patients represents an important area of work as our population ages and as geriatric patients are often not included at the same rate as younger patients in clinical trials.[148,149]

Gender Effects

There is still a lot to learn about the effects of gender on drug pharmacokinetics and pharmacodynamics. However, we are briefly highlighting here some important differences that have emerged in recent meta-analyses or data pooled from Phase 3 trials. For example, a recent meta-analysis suggests that women have a greater incidence of the potentially traumatic experience of awareness under general anesthesia, while also emerging more quickly from anesthesia than men.[150] Recent meta-analysis also shows that women receiving treatment for schizophrenia have a higher response to antipsychotic medication than men, with the number needed to treat (NNT) for a response in women being 6.9 and the NNT for men being 9.4.[151] Based on data from Phase 3 clinical trials, it also appears that women experience greater improvements in lipid levels after treatment with bempedoic acid, compared to men.[152]

Genetic Variation

One of the most common sources of differences in individual response to drug therapy is genetic variation in genes encoding proteins needed in drug metabolism and effect. Consider, for example, probably the most commonly used drug in the world: caffeine. Variation in the CYP1A2 gene (specifically, those who are homozygous or heterozygous for the -163C>A polymorphism) is an important contributing factor to the rate at which caffeine is metabolized.[153] When combined with other factors that can affect caffeine availability, such as differences in the rate of gastric emptying, the result is considerable variability in how long it takes for caffeine to reach its maximum levels in the bloodstream. This can take as little as 20 minutes but can also take up to 120 minutes when someone consumes a cup of hot coffee, and the range is larger, 20 to 240 minutes, when someone consumes a cold energy drink.[154] Moreover, while an average half-life (the time for an active amount of drug in the body to be reduced by half) for caffeine is four to six hours, the range of half-life is also of considerable magnitude, from two to twelve hours.[155] In essence, by the time some people reach peak blood levels, active caffeine levels may already be reduced by half in others!

As diabetes is now estimated to affect about 1 in 10 Americans, and 90% to 95% of these roughly thirty-eight million people in the United

States are diagnosed with type 2 diabetes,[156] we feel it is important to review some of the pharmacogenetic factors impacting the treatment of this common condition. Several genetic variants are suggested to impact the pharmacokinetics or dynamics of drugs commonly used in treating type 2 diabetes. For example, a study of 478 patients taking metformin found that those carrying or homozygous for the "G" allele of the SLC22A1 gene variant rs628031 G/A (a gene encoding a cation transporter[157]) showed increased likelihood to be responders to metformin monotherapy.[158]

Another gene variant of significant import is the G972R mutation of the insulin receptor substrate-1 gene. This variant results in a glycine to arginine substitution at codon 972 and is present in about 10% of those with type 2 diabetes and around 6% of the general population.[159] This variant is associated with reduced insulin sensitivity[160] and an increased risk of treatment failure with oral antidiabetic drugs;[161] it also has been reported to be a significant independent predictor of coronary heart disease,[162] which is an important consideration given the overlap of type 2 diabetes and heart disease. Also important in the context of heart disease and diabetes is an effect of a mutation in the 5' region of the PROX1 gene (a gene enabling transcription factor activity and shaping organ development[163]), the single-nucleotide polymorphism (SNP) known as rs340874, which is a potential risk factor for hyperglycemia due to use of atenolol.[164]

Finally, it may be especially important to consider the presence of polymorphisms of the CYP2C9 gene, needed for sulfonylurea metabolism, in elderly subjects with type 2 diabetes receiving treatment with sulfonylurea drugs. In a study that included 103 subjects over the age of sixty, the rate of hypoglycemic episodes increased according to the number of polymorphisms present for the CYP2CP gene. Over three months, those with two wild-type alleles experienced 0.36±0.98 episodes (mean±SD), those with one polymorphism experienced 0.79±1.7 episodes, and those with two polymorphisms experienced 2.67±4.6 episodes.[165]

Given the impact of the ongoing opioid epidemic, we also discuss briefly some pharmacogenetic differences that impact the effectiveness of opioid drugs. Opioid pain treatment is an area where patients exhibit significant individual variability in response. For example, one study in cancer patients showed that while most patients responded to morphine, about 25% did not, and most of these did respond when changed to an alternative opioid.[166] While no single genetic difference explains this variation, several genetic variants are beginning to emerge as important contributing factors. Among these is the SNP in the μ-opioid receptor gene known as A118G, in which there is an aspartate substitution for asparagine at position 40. A structural impact of this substitution is the removal of an N-glycosylation site in the receptor, which while not affecting the binding of the receptor to opioid alkaloids, may increase its affinity for the endogenous ligand, β-endorphin.[167]

The results of a meta-analysis of twenty-three studies (Ren 2015) suggest that the presence of this allele is associated with higher pain scores in the first twenty-four hours of the postoperative period, as well as greater opioid consumption and a reduced risk of vomiting. Thus, the overall picture suggests a somewhat reduced sensitivity to the effects of opioids in patients with this SNP.[168] This view is reinforced by a recent update of the analysis, expanded to include thirty-nine studies and 7,455 patients.[169] This expanded analysis confirms that patients carrying the A118G allele, which occurs in about 16% of Northern and Western Europeans and 46.5% in Asians, required greater levels of opioids in the first twenty-four hours after surgery. In addition to evidence showing that this allele affects sensitivity to opioid medications, there is also evidence from an observational study that its presence is associated with significantly increased risk of severe clinical outcomes (respiratory/cardiac arrest) in cases of overdose [OR:5.3, 95% CI, 1.2-23.8, P < 0.05].[170]

In addition to highlighting the importance of the A118G polymorphism, the previously cited updated analysis (Li 2023) was also able to detect a difference associated with the CYP3A4*1G variant, which leads to a single G-to-A substitution resulting in reduced function of the CYP3A4 metabolizing enzyme. Those carrying the CYP3A4*1G variant required smaller doses of opioids in the first twenty-four hours after surgery compared to those not carrying the variant. As reviewed by the authors of the analysis, this is a high-frequency allele in Asians (0.249 in Japanese and 0.221 in Chinese).

To further inform clinicians about the known impacts of genetic variations on the most commonly prescribed drugs, we have cross-referenced information in FDA's table of pharmacogenetic biomarkers and associated drug labeling text with a list of frequently prescribed drugs. This effort aims to provide a concise summary of some of the most vital pharmacogenetic information from FDA's table for drugs that are among the fifty most commonly prescribed.

Cross-Reference of FDA's Table of Pharmacogenetic Biomarkers in Drug Labeling with List of Commonly Prescribed Drugs

Drug	Pharmacogenetic biomarker	Summary of key pharmacogenetic relevance found in drug labeling
Omeprazole (proton pump inhibitor)	CYP2C19	A person is an extensive, intermediate, or "poor metabolizer"*[173] depending on the number of functional alleles that are present for CYP2C19. At steady state, poor metabolizers have 1.5 times the level of the rest of the population, but this change is not considered clinically meaningful.
Metoprolol (beta-blocker)	CYP2D6	Metoprolol is metabolized predominantly by CYP2D6, which, when inhibited by several drugs (such as quinidine and propafenone) can lead to a several-fold increase in metoprolol levels and thus increase risk of adverse effects outside of the heart tissue. In addition, CYP2D6 is absent in about 8% of Caucasians and about 2% of most other populations. Those with absent CYP2D6 are poor metabolizers of the drug.
Fluoxetine (antidepressant: selective serotonin reuptake inhibitor)	CYP2D6	Fluoxetine is an inhibitor of CYP2D6 and may make those with normal CYP2D6 function resemble poor metabolizers. This may explain the association between fluoxetine use and risk of QT interval prolongation and ventricular arrhythmias, as CYP2D6 inhibitors predispose to this adverse effect.
Citalopram (antidepressant: selective serotonin reuptake inhibitor)	CYP2C19	In CYP2C19 poor metabolizers the AUC is increased by 107%. Due to risk of QT prolongation, the maximum dose of citalopram (Celexa) in poor CYP2C19 metabolizers is 20 mg/d.

Bupropion (antidepressant: inhibits reuptake of dopamine and norepinephrine)	CYP2D6	Bupropion and its metabolites are CYP2D6 inhibitors and have been shown to increase the AUC of desipramine in extensive metabolizers of CYP2C19 fivefold. The effects of increasing desipramine were seen for at least seven days after the last dose of bupropion.
Carvedilol (beta-blocker)	CYP2D6	Poor metabolizers of CYP2D6 have two- to threefold higher plasma concentrations of the (R+) enantiomer of carvedilol and a 20 to 25% increase in the levels of carvedilol (S+) enantiomer. During up-titration of dose, poor metabolizers of CYP2D6 had increased rates of dizziness.
Tramadol (opioid analgesic)	CYP2D6	Those who are ultrarapid metabolizers of CYP2D6 experience increased exposure to tramadol's active metabolite, O-desmethyltramadol, created by the action of CYP2D6. This can lead to life-threatening respiratory depression and signs of overdose, including sleepiness, confusion, and shallow breathing. The genotype associated with ultrarapid metabolizers is estimated to be present in 1 to 10% of Whites, 3 to 4% of Blacks, 1 to 2% of East Asians, and may be greater than 10% in Oceanian, Northern African, and Middle Eastern people, as well as Ashkenazi Jews and Puerto Ricans.

Pantoprazole (proton pump inhibitor)	CYP2C19	About 3% of Caucasians and African-Americans and 17 to 23% of East Asians are poor metabolizers of CYP2C19 due to genetic polymorphism. For adults, this may lead to half lives of three-and-a-half to ten hours, though with minimal accumulation, no change in dosing is needed. In children, poor metabolizers may have oral clearance that is tenfold less than rapid metabolizers, and in this population, dose reduction should be considered.
Rosuvastatin (statin)	SLCO1B1 (gene encoding the OATP1B1 transporter)	Those with the polymorphism SLCO1B1 521 C/C have poor functioning of two alleles encoding for the OATP1B1 transporter and have increased levels of rosuvastatin. This polymorphism is reported to generally exist in less than 5% of most racial groups, and its impacts of efficacy and safety have not been clearly established.
Meloxicam (NSAID)	CYP2C9	Meloxicam AUC is substantially higher in those with reduced CYP2C activity, especially in those who are poor metabolizers. The frequency of poor metabolizer genotypes is present in < 5% of the population. In patients known or suspected to be poor CYP2C9 metabolizers based on genetic testing or previous experience with other CYP2C9 substrates (e.g., warfarin or phenytoin), health care professionals should consider dose reduction.

Clopidogrel (antiplatelet drug)	CYP2C19	The action of clopidogrel (Plavix) depends on the creation of an active metabolite, mainly through the action of CYP2C19. Those who are homozygous for nonfunctional alleles of CYP2C19 are poor metabolizers and show decreased exposure to the active metabolite and diminished inhibition of platelet aggregation. The genotype leading to poor metabolism is found in about 2% of White patients, 4% of Black patients, and 14% of Chinese patients.
Glipizide (sulfonylurea, antidiabetic drug)	G6PD	Sulfonylurea agents such as glipizide can lead to hemolytic anemia in patients with G6PD deficiency. This finding has been additionally reported in some patients who did not have G6PD deficiency.
Warfarin (anticoagulant)	CYP2C9	The S-enantiomer of warfarin is metabolized mainly by CYP2C9. Two variant alleles, CYP2C9*2 and CYP2C9*3, lead to decreased hydroxylation of S-warfarin, in vitro. The frequency of the CYP2C9*2 allele is approximately 11% and that of CYP2C9*3 is about 7% in Caucasians. Other CYP2C9 alleles also associated with reduced enzymatic activity occur at lesser frequencies. Warfarin hinders vitamin K regeneration via VKOR inhibition. Specific VKORC1 gene variants, such as -1639G>A, affect warfarin dosing.

Tamsulosin (alpha-1 blocker used to treat enlarged prostate)	CYP2D6	It is known that using a strong CYP2D6 inhibitor like paroxetine concurrently increases the AUC of tamsulosin (Flomax) by 1.6 times. It is therefore expected that poor metabolizers of CYP2D6 would exhibit similarly elevated levels, comparing poor metabolizers to extensive metabolizers. About 7% of Caucasians are poor metabolizers, as are about 2% of African Americans.
Duloxetine (antidepressant: serotonin-nor-adrenaline re-uptake inhibitor)	CYP2D6	When CYP2D6 poor metabolizers were given a CYP1A2 inhibitor (fluvoxamine) along with duloxetine, a sixfold increase in the AUC of duloxetine was seen.

Sources: FDA's Table of Pharmacogenetic Biomarkers in Drug Labeling[171] with List of Commonly Prescribed Drugs[172]

It is worth underscoring that both inhibition and induction of differing hepatic enzymes can have toxic effects depending on the drug that is being metabolized. For example, fluoxetine, which inhibits CYP2D6 function, can cause the QT interval (the time it takes for the ventricles to contract and relax again) to lengthen, increasing the potential for dangerous ventricular arrhythmias, while excessive induction of the same enzyme can lead to toxic levels of tramadol's active metabolite and increased risk of respiratory depression.

In addition to awareness of estimates of drug effect reported in human studies, practitioners benefit when their prescribing decisions for an individual are informed by consideration of the patient's unique characteristics, as we have argued. In addition to considering a patient's existing list of medications to screen for interactions, it is also important not to lose sight of other key factors that shape the patient's unique response. These include the effects of preexisting inflammation, the reduced hepatic and renal blood flow that accompanies aging, and the presence of potentially impactful genetic variants. Diligence in identifying these factors—and in the case of inflammation, addressing this factor to the extent possible—may lead to improved efficiency and predictability of an individual's response to pharmacotherapy or at least make the clinician more aware of when especially close monitoring is needed.

Now that we have delved into a good deal of background on how drugs are dosed and why predicting individual response, including adverse events, is so difficult, it's time to return to the issue of drug safety that we raised earlier in this book as we consider the question "how well-defined are toxicity curves before drug approval?" This is an opportunity to appreciate with greater depth what is going wrong in our drug approval process and to understand why the principle of low-dose combination therapy inherent in traditional herbal medicine is needed now more than ever.

CHAPTER 7

How Well-Defined are Toxicity Curves Before Drug Approval?

Historical Context

To improve FDA's ability to evaluate new drug applications, Congress passed the Prescription Drug User Fee Act in 1992.[174] This act allows FDA to charge fees to pharmaceutical companies, providing the agency with the resources it needs for application reviews. However, this funding model has the unintended consequence of making FDA see drug companies, rather than the general public, as their primary client (see epilogue for more information to this point).

In 1994, in issuing its guidance to industry about which study designs should be utilized to gather dose-response data moving forward, the International Conference on Harmonisation of Technical Requirements for the Registration of Pharmaceuticals for Human Use (ICH) assessed the inherent difficulties of trying to adequately derive dose-response data by stating, in part:[175]

Historically, marketers have often initially presented drugs as treatments later recognized as excessive doses (i.e., doses well onto the plateau of the dose-response curve for the desired effect), sometimes with adverse consequences (e.g., hypokalemia and other metabolic disturbances with thiazide-type diuretics in hypertension). This situation has been improved by attempts to find the smallest dose with a discernible useful effect or a maximum dose beyond which no further beneficial effect is seen, but practical study designs do not exist to allow for precise determination of these doses. Further, expanding knowledge indicates that the concepts of minimum effective dose and maximum useful dose do not adequately account for individual differences and do not allow a comparison, at various doses, of both beneficial and undesirable effects. Any given dose provides a mixture of desirable and undesirable effects, with no single dose necessarily optimal for all patients.

Even though the ICH has highlighted shortcomings in dose-response research, and despite FDA having more resources to more fully evaluate drug applications, the safety of FDA-approved drugs hasn't improved. In 2014 researchers estimated that since 1992, about a quarter of newly approved drugs (26.7 per 100 drugs) received a black box warning or underwent market withdrawal after approval. The rate before 1992 was 21.2 per 100 drugs, indicating that drugs approved after the Prescription Drug User Fee Act are more likely to have serious safety problems than drugs approved before the 1992 act.[176]

While there is probably more than one simple reason for the lack of progress in preventing postmarket safety problems with approved drugs, we feel we must ask, if even with helpful guidance to improve dose-response data gathering and greater regulatory resources to evaluate drug safety, the rate of safety concerns remains high (or even increases), do we not have a fundamental problem with unsafe drugs entering the marketplace?

Closing the Information Gap in Dosing

One of the roots of this problem is the often significant gap between the dose of a drug that produces a desired response in half the population, ED_{50}, and the actual dose of drugs approved and then prescribed in the marketplace, an issue partly addressed in chapter 3. A further example of the dilemma caused by the delta between ED_{50} and doses used in practice is the case of aspirin when used to prevent cardiovascular disease over recent decades. Since the late 1980s, health care professionals have commonly recommended aspirin to prevent various forms of cardiovascular disease,[177] with ensuing FDA approval.[178] However, it has taken decades for a more mature understanding of the relatively small benefit and the risk of bleeding to be fully appreciated.[179] Authorities have approved doses as high as 1,300 mg per day (mg/d) in the US; however, doses as low as 30 mg/d are shown to fully inhibit platelet thromboxane production.[180]

While a more reasonable dose of 81 mg/d has recently been the most commonly used dose, in the 2000s, a dose of 325 mg/d still represented the second-most widely used dose in 35% of cases.[181] This is unfortunate as data from observational studies do not support any increase in efficacy beyond 75 to 81mg/d, while larger doses show an increase in the risk of bleeding.[182] If it has taken this long to really articulate the trade-offs in benefit and safety along the dose-response curve for something as common as aspirin, how much do we know about the safety of other modern medicines? How carefully are effect and safety titrated in newly approved drugs?

While we, like everyone, probably have a whole lot to learn about the safety profile of drugs now on the market, one positive step might be to simply require drug marketing advertisements and prescribing information provided to patients through pharmacies to disclose any available ED_{50} for the prescribed use and the context of what ED_{50} (the dose that achieves a desired effect in half the population) means. How different would the conversation be between patient and provider if truly informed patients asked, "Why do I need to take a dose so much above the ED_{50}?" If prescribers don't actually know all the safety nuances of use at doses well onto the plateau of the dose-response curve, why, except in cases where only maximal and immediate benefits are needed to save a patient's life, would one want to start with aggressive dosing?

Another challenge contributing to the ambiguity in clinical decision-making stems from the reality articulated in the ICH statement: "There are variations among individuals determining how well a drug works and how much harm it causes at any particular dose." While dose-response data better bring into focus the central tendency of data gathered from a population, differences in genes encoding for drug-metabolizing enzymes, variations in body size and composition, diet, microbiome composition, and other concurrent medication use are among the factors that may affect the pharmacokinetics and pharmacodynamics of a drug. The statistics generally used to describe dose responses are usually applied to data from a population, not an individual. However, it is the unique response of any given patient that really matters at the moment that they are the focus of clinical care: odds of what adverse events may or may not occur in a population are eclipsed by any catastrophic outcome that occurs with 100% reality in a single individual.

Moreover, the signal-to-noise ratio can change as one moves from lower to higher doses. Specifically, less immediately life-threatening toxicities, especially those that may manifest when starting a drug and then wane in the short term, are more difficult to identify at lower doses than severe toxic effects that occur more quickly at larger doses. With relatively lower signal and higher noise at lower doses, it is difficult to determine when toxicity first really begins to declare itself. Also, while it is financially advantageous to structure a study with as few subjects as necessary to see an effect tied to efficacy, there is no guarantee that a study with enough power to detect a desired effect will also have enough subjects to detect the most important safety signals. Larger studies reduce the chance of statistical error of missing a relevant toxicity effect. A more balanced approach in study design would be to power studies to detect *both* an outcome of efficacy and, at the very least, what can be anticipated as the most likely or concerning adverse events.

Given the mix of both desirable and undesirable effects at any given dose studied in a population and the changes in signal-to-noise ratio that exist along any dose-response curve, perhaps those trying to precisely predict an optimal dose for an individual patient may wish to temporarily change places with physicists attempting to pinpoint the exact location of any given particle and then frankly discuss which is the more fruitful of the two exercises.

The Variable of Time

While what we have written above clarifies some of the real challenges confronting drug usage in the United States and the world, this should not be interpreted as a blanket indictment of the marketers' motives. There has to be room to learn new things about drugs. Aspirin, a drug on the market for many years, was later found to have some additional, though perhaps modest, action in reducing the risk of cardiovascular disease. That's a good thing. But if in our need to quickly address a pressing health concern we intervene without knowing as much as possible about safety trade-offs, then we need a strong system to flesh out the more complete safety picture over time.

Currently, the FDA requires or initiates various postmarketing studies when a drug or biologic is approved. These studies include postmarketing requirements (PMRs), which are mandatory, and postmarketing commitments (PMCs), which are voluntary commitments made by the drug company. In fact, about 80% of newly approved therapeutics (both drugs and biologics) must perform at least one clinical study, which about 60% of the time takes the form of a prospective cohort study, registry, or clinical trial.[183] This is good progress in terms of the number of current studies. However, most drugs are approved based on several studies of up to only a few years each, and some adverse effects may only manifest after five-plus years of use, so we reiterate the previously noted observation that a critical factor of postmarketing studies is the length of time of these studies.[184]

To illustrate just how critical the variable of time is to determine drug safety, we highlight the work of the DAD study group, which, in a prospective observational study of over 20,000 patients with HIV, found that the incidence of myocardial infarction for those taking protease inhibitors over six years was 6.01 per 1,000 person-years, while for those patients not exposed to protease inhibitors, the incidence was 1.53 per 1,000 person-years.[185] Conducting such a long-term prospective study was crucial for uncovering this important information, which would have otherwise gone unnoticed. In understanding drug safety, studying a drug for a longer duration often reveals its unique qualities.

Due to the pragmatic challenges of prospective clinical trials done over this length of time, such as patients wanting to try different medications or not wanting to take a placebo for many years, it makes sense to uniformly require that after drugs obtain approval, they be monitored in a prospective observation study for at least seven years to more fully identify the risk of adverse effects. This active approach would greatly increase the safety data collected in conjunction with the passive reporting currently collected by submitting reports through the MedWatch system.

Of course, we cannot help but point out that with a more complete picture of the longer-term safety of newly-approved, single drugs being elusive, low-dose combination therapy will at some point come to be clearly understood as the superior approach for long-term safety as well. This is because combining medicines in lower doses buffers the toxicity of any single agent. As "the dose makes the poison," give a lower dose whenever possible!

As critical as the concern of safety is, there is also opportunity to exploit the therapeutic benefit of low-dose combination therapy; after all, medicines need to work in order to be useful, as well as being safe. This potential is highlighted as we consider a concept long-revered in herbal medicine that should also be more utilized in conventional pharmacology: synergy.

CHAPTER 8

Combination Therapy as a Cauldron for Synergy

Understanding Synergy in Medicine

One of the most fascinating aspects of combination therapy is the potential for a combination of medicinal ingredients to have a synergistic effect. Practitioners of many kinds, and perhaps especially naturopathic physicians, rightly have a great affection for the term "synergism" because it alludes to maximizing benefit by bringing together the best-fitting combination of available ingredients to fill a patient's needs. But what exactly do we mean when we speak of synergy?

This chapter more clearly defines synergy, explores how synergy occurs in combination therapy, and suggests ways in which a traditional approach to combination botanical therapy can facilitate this phenomenon.

What Does Synergy Mean?

As reviewed by Breitinger,[186] the word "synergy" is derived from the Greek term *synergos*, which means "to work together" and suggests that "the combination and interaction of two or more agents or forces with a combined effect that is greater than the sum of their individual effects." We would counsel a slightly rephrased working definition: synergy is a combination of effect interactions that leads to a greater impact than the sum of individual effects.

To clarify the meaning of synergy, comparing and contrasting synergistic effects with additive effects is also helpful. Additive effects are those that have no interaction with each other at all.[187] Thus synergy is when interactions create a greater overall impact than occurs without interactions. At the same time, individual effects that are free from interactions with each other are better described as additive, meaning they add independently to create whatever turns out to be the overall impact. It might be clarifying, in fact, to refer to additive effects as simply noninteractive effects. And, in truth, when one considers the broad potential for ingredients to interact in unforeseen ways across complex body systems, it might be the case that truly additive effects, in vivo, are rare exceptions and synergistic interactions are more common than is generally realized. There are many ways that a synergistic effect can be achieved, including interactions that affect how a medicine moves through the body (absorption, distribution, metabolism, and excretion—pharmacokinetics) and interactions that affect how a medicine acts on the body (pharmacodynamics).

Formulation philosophies centered in combination therapy facilitate synergy, not just because multiple botanicals are combined but because there are intentional roles of ingredients that formulators seek to fill when formulating medicines.

Synergistic Interactions—Traditional and Modern

In traditional Chinese medicine (TCM), herbs are often combined in a specific manner to achieve maximum therapeutic effectiveness. The formula typically includes four types of herbs: a "monarch" herb that serves as the main active ingredient, a "minister" herb that enhances the effects of the monarch, an "assistant" herb that reduces any potential side effects or toxicity, and a "guide" herb that helps deliver all the other herbs more efficiently to targeted areas in the body.[188] When one adds an assistant herb to minimize the toxicity of the monarch herb, the entire formula becomes both safer and more effective than using just the monarch herb on its own. Similarly, suppose a minister herb interacts with the monarch herb in favorably affecting pharmacodynamics at a target receptor. In that case, the therapeutic effect may be better than if the minister or monarch herb were given alone. Lastly, even if a guide herb doesn't offer much therapeutic value by itself, it may improve the pharmacokinetics of delivery of the monarch and minister herbs to the point that the combination has significantly more action at a target site.

Historically, Western scientists have often dismissed this TCM model as anthropomorphic magical thinking. This is not the case; the labels simply help to define and communicate how the various herbs are intended to work together to accomplish a desired result. Studying the effects of some of the individual herbs and their combinations can illustrate the power of the TCM combinatorial model. We will use this analogy of herbs with different functions from TCM when describing examples of synergistic combinations below, whether or not the examples specifically originate from a TCM formula.

A simple example of herbal synergism that occurs with monarch and minister herbs manifests in studying the traditional formula, Shuan-long, which is composed of *Panax ginseng* and *Salvia miltiorrhiza*, with *Panax* being the more abundant herb in the formulation. Comparing the effect of the individual ingredients of the traditional formula to their combination in a rat model of myocardial infarction, a synergistic improvement in efficacy was found.[189] Specifically, the model showed the herbal combination to intensify the ability of rats to recover normal energetic metabolism after an MI, and while each herb helped protect cardiac muscle to a degree from necrosis, neither herb was equally as protective as the combination. Both herbs in this example show some effect by themselves that is not equal to their effect when combined.

A modern example of how principles of combination therapy can lead to synergism using monarch and assistant ingredients is found in recent research examining the effects of combining the chemotherapy drug 5-fluorouracil (5-FU) with a Chinese medicine Bu-Zhong-Yi-Qi (itself an herbal combination of ten different herbs).[190] Administering this chemotherapy-herbal combination to mice injected with murine gastric cancer cells significantly increased the survival time of mice receiving the chemotherapy-herbal combination relative to mice receiving the chemotherapy drug by itself. This was in spite of the fact that the tumor-inhibiting action of the herbs by themselves was much less than that exhibited by 5FU by itself. In humans given the same chemotherapy drug or drug-plus-herbs, it was also observed that those receiving the combination versus the drug alone had a significantly lower proportion of CD8+PD-1+ cells. As PD-1 expression is a compensatory response known to be induced by the chemotherapy drug that allows some cancer cells to escape immune detection, in this instance, the entire herbal combination is acting as the assistant to help offset the toxicity of the monarch chemotherapy drug, with a good indication of synergy (the prolonged survival seen in the evaluable animal data).

Another important example of synergism, and an example of a guide ingredient producing synergism in combination with a monarch ingredient, is the combination of an active from one of the traditional Ayurvedic medicines, Trikatu, and poorly absorbed curcumin. Using a rat model of depression induced by chronic stress, piperine, an active of the black and long pepper in Trikatu, is given in conjunction with curcumin. Curcumin's ability to decrease immobility and restore brain neurotransmitter levels is significantly enhanced compared to the effects seen with curcumin alone.[191] Importantly, researchers applied the synergistic combination of curcumin and piperine, as demonstrated in basic science work, to enhance clinical efficacy in a sizeable clinical trial as an adjunctive treatment for depression.[192] As a combination of bioavailability enhancers, the piperine-containing peppers of Trikatu and its gingerol-providing ginger may be one of the superior synergizing formulas refined over its long period of empirical use. This is in part because both ingredients enhance the surface area of the absorptive surface and increase its membrane fluidity, while also potentially slowing biotransformation pathways (Phase I, Phase II, and p-glycoprotein action).[193,194,195,196,197,198] Moreover, gingerol is known to increase mineral absorption (sodium) through TRPV1 agonism, a receptor also known to be agonized by piperazine.[199,200]

Delightfully, positive synergistic interactions that are quite unanticipated can also occur (as can negative interactions that professionals should screen for and exclude whenever possible). For instance, sometimes a medicine that we think is only an assistant used to offset adverse effects also has some minister effects. An example: when N-acetylcysteine (NAC) is used to antidote acetaminophen's hepatotoxicity, NAC can also exert an analgesic effect in concert with acetaminophen, as measured with the hot plate test in rats.[201] By the way, is there any good reason manufacturers don't already include NAC as a co-ingredient in acetaminophen (beyond FDA regulations)?

When including herbal ingredients to fill roles in formulation, predicting all their interactions is impossible. However, both centuries of empirical observation and modern research have helped us identify many positive interactions between herbs and to harness these interactions for clinical benefit. At the same time, this reality does not to any degree diminish the need for the time careful pharmacists and clinicians invest to avoid detrimental interactions, which is critical to promote safety. It rather points to the fact that in addition to identifying and preventing negative interactions wherever possible, we should also seek to maximize beneficial synergistic interactions to provide the best possible intervention.

CHAPTER 9

Drug-Herb Interactions Shown in Human Data

We have explored a wealth of scientific insights that can guide safer use of both herbal and conventional medicines. With these principles outlined, our discussion would be incomplete without delving into the crucial specifics of how herbs, foods, and drugs interact within the body. The following two chapters offer key reference information on this topic, drawing from the latest available scientific literature.

There are many ways that herbs and prescription drugs can affect the movement (kinetics) and effects (dynamics) of each other in the body. This includes changes in how each is absorbed, metabolized by enzymes in the liver and other organs, and excreted through the kidneys and bowels, as well as how they interact with receptors that mediate their effects. People often focus on unwanted herbal-drug interactions when they perceive an herb as interfering with a drug's desired effects. However, it is equally correct to state that a prescription drug may interfere with a well-applied herbal medicine. Moreover, an optimal evaluation of a drug or an herb's safety profile should consider the context of an individual patient's diet. Some drugs may have varying safety issues that arise when diets change. For example, when dietary intake of vitamin K exceeds about 150 mcg/d, it can significantly alter the safety profile of the anticoagulant drug warfarin; therefore, a suggested strategy for reducing the risk of mishaps with warfarin dosing is to carefully maintain a consistent level of vitamin K intake in the diet.[202]

Most of the data collected to date and available for review speak to known interactions of an herb altering aspects of a drug's action. Since such interactions may lead to catastrophic clinical outcomes, we focus on these data in our review. However, it's both right and fair to say that when using a reasonable course of herbal medicine, one should also be aware of any potential interference from conventional medicines.

This field is rich in in vitro data indicating possible adverse interactions and in vivo animal studies that inform pharmacist and practitioner guidelines. Yet human clinical data, which hold the most significance, is scarcer. This review focuses on human studies and case reports to highlight clear, applicable interaction evidence. Typically, we've analyzed interactions by individual herbs. For analgesics and anti-inflammatories, however, grouping the data provides a clearer overview.

Analgesics (Pain Relievers / Anti-Inflammatories)

Some of the most common pain relievers used are the analgesic acetaminophen and the nonsteroidal anti-inflammatory drugs, such as ibuprofen. One of the herbs most commonly studied for its anti-inflammatory effects is *Curcumin longa* (turmeric), whose main actives, the curcuminoids, are often administered with small amounts of piperine (a constituent of black pepper) to enhance their absorption.

A randomized, controlled crossover study of eight subjects examined the effect of several days of pretreatment with curcuminoids and piperine on the pharmacokinetics of acetaminophen and a drug closely related to ibuprofen (flurbiprofen). In this study, short-term pretreatment with curcuminoids and piperine did not show any effects on the pharmacokinetics of acetaminophen or flurbiprofen.[203] As noted by the authors, these findings are in contrast to in vitro work from the same team.[204] Although the results did not provide evidence of an interaction with typical curcuminoid extract over the short term, we highlight these results as they provide an important opportunity to understand better why in vitro results that suggest an interaction do not necessarily correlate with human results.

In this case, the authors point out that the in vivo levels of curcuminoids are relatively low compared with levels that lead to changes in the activity of drug-metabolizing enzymes in vitro. Moreover, the curcuminoids detectable in vivo in this study are mostly conjugated (through glucuronidation or sulfation), and thus, the potential for these conjugated forms to affect drug metabolism is not known. It may be that any effect of curcuminoids on drug-metabolizing enzymes is a dynamic heavily affected by the rate of curcuminoid absorption and how efficiently curcuminoid conjugation is taking place in the gut and/or liver. In vivo, realities of absorption and biotransformation occurring closely in tandem exemplify how complex environments that can be mimicked to only a limited degree during in vitro testing make translation of basic science research to real-world scenarios challenging.

One of Korea's most frequently used herbal medicine combinations is known as Ojeok-san. From 1990 to 2010, it represented the most commonly used herbal medicine supplied by the National Health Insurance Corporation of Korea. Among its many uses is that of an analgesic.[205] Its formula is composed of small amounts of seventeen herbs in combination, including mandarin orange peel (*Citrus reticulata Blanco*), ginger root, jujube fruit, licorice root, and Chinese peony root, among others.[206] In a study involving twenty human subjects, taking Ojeok-san and the common anti-inflammatory drug celecoxib together showed a trend toward reduced maximum and total blood concentrations (C_{max} and AUC) of celecoxib compared to taking celecoxib alone. Additionally, the combination of Ojeok-san and celecoxib tended to slow down the rate of celecoxib elimination.[207] The present data do not inform us how the potential changes in the kinetics of celecoxib may ultimately impact its effectiveness as a pain reliever.

To cite another example, one of the most common drugs used to treat neuropathic pain is gabapentin. In terms of dietary-drug interactions, there is an interesting, albeit not necessarily clinically impactful, interaction between gabapentin and shitake, a mushroom consumed in the diet (and consumed also in dietary supplements). In healthy subjects, dietary shitake mushroom slightly increased the renal clearance of gabapentin, though this change was not enough to significantly alter the in vivo concentration (area under the concentration time curve, or AUC) of gabapentin.[208]

Goldenseal

There is evidence from a human study that in acting as an inhibitor of the drug-metabolizing enzyme CYP3A4, goldenseal increases the in vivo concentration of the benzodiazepine drug midazolam (increased AUC, as well as maximum serum concentration, C_{max}), while slowing its rate of clearance.[209] Additional work in healthy humans shows that goldenseal decreases the metabolism of the drug debrisoquine, a drug used as a marker for CYP2D6 activity.[210] Further, a human study shows that goldenseal lowers the AUC of metformin.[211] Researchers have also evaluated goldenseal in humans for its potential to influence activity of the cellular drug transporter p–glycoprotein, using digoxin as a marker of p-glycoprotein action, not finding evidence of an observable effect on this important aspect of drug metabolism.[212] This illustrates that a single herb may impact drug metabolism through multiple mechanisms, so effects often cannot be predicted by a single action.

Salvia miltiorrhiza

One of the medicines used in China to improve circulation in cases of heart disease is an extract of the plant *Salvia miltiorrhiza*. When combined with aspirin, this herbal medicine produces some interesting effects on the kinetics of both actives identified in the plant extract and salicylic acid, the active of aspirin. One of the herbal actives, salvianolic acid B, has both a longer elimination time and a decrease in its total concentration (AUC) when taken with aspirin. The body absorbs salicylic acid more quickly and in smaller amounts with the herbal extract of *Salvia miltiorrhiza* present. However, researchers still need to determine how these differences in absorption affect the clinical effectiveness of the extract and aspirin.

St. John's Wort

Perhaps no other herb is as extensively studied for its potential to interact with drugs as St. John's wort. At present, most of the information on this herb is in the context of its ability to increase both the expression of a liver enzyme that metabolizes many drugs (CYP3A4) and to increase the activity of the drug transporter p-glycoprotein, which removes many drugs from a cell's interior. The combined effects of CYP3A4 induction and increased p-glycoprotein activity underscore the relatively high potential for St. John's wort to lower in vivo levels of drugs, thus potentially leading to changes in pharmacodynamics. Zhou has extensively reviewed prescription drugs that have reduced blood levels when taken with St. John's wort.[213] These findings, as well as those from several additional sources identified in the literature, are summarized below:

Drugs levels reduced by concurrent use with St. John's wort, based on human data

Drug interacting with St. John's wort	Effect reported	Category of human data
Amitriptyline	Lower blood concentration	Clinical study[214]
Cyclosporine	Lower blood concentration	Case report[215]
Digoxin	Lower blood concentration	Clinical study[216]
Fexofenadine	Lower blood concentration	Clinical study[217]
Gliclazide	Lower blood concentration	Clinical study[218]
Indinavir	Lower blood concentration	Clinical study[219]
Methadone	Lower blood concentration	Clinical study[220]
Midazolam	Lower blood concentration	Clinical study[221]
Nevirapine	Lower blood concentration	Case series (n=5)[222]
Oxycodone	Lower blood concentration	Clinical study[223]
Phenprocoumon	Lower blood concentration	Clinical study[224]
Simvastatin	Lower blood concentration	Clinical study[225]
Tacrolimus	Lower blood concentration	Clinical study[226]
Theophylline	Lower blood concentration	Case report[227]
Warfarin	Lower blood concentration	Case series (n=7)[228]; clinical study[229], clinical study[230]

It can be difficult to anticipate if a particular herb-drug interaction might exist based on interaction data from a drug in the same category or even based on a single known action on biotransforming enzymes. An example is the current differing data regarding interactions between St. John's wort and fentanyl and St. John's wort and oxycodone. In the case of St. John's wort and fentanyl, there was no pharmacokinetic or pharmacodynamic interaction when human subjects consumed 900 mg of St. John's wort extract over thirty days and also received fentanyl infusions, nor were there any significant effects on fentanyl's analgesic effects.[231] This finding contrasts the demonstrated interaction between St. John's wort and oxycodone noted above. Even though CYP3A4 and p-glycoprotein affect the metabolism of many drugs (CYP3A4, for example, is estimated to affect the metabolism of over half of known drugs because of the low specificity with which it binds to substrates[232]), the effect of CYP3A4 is also dependent on genetic polymorphisms of CYP3A4.[233] Additionally, while induction of CYP3A4 is a predominant effect, there seem to be inhibitory effects of St. John's wort constituents on other CYP (P450) enzymes.[234] Thus, the overall interaction of St. John's wort (and likely many other herbs) with any given drug depends on the sum effects of multiple biotransformation aspects. Given the noted disparity that can also occur between results from in vitro / animal testing and human testing, we feel it necessary to stress again that applicable human data is a potent, though relatively rare, clarifier in the sphere of herb-drug interaction data.

Green Tea

If St. John's wort is the most studied herb for its interactions with drugs, the catechins from green tea may be a strong second, with multiple human studies accumulating in the last few years. The human data on this topic includes a 2017 open-label study of thirteen healthy subjects finding that coadministration of a single dose of 300 mg epigallocatechin-3-gallate (EGCG) with 20 mg of rosuvastatin resulted in a significant decrease in rosuvastatin's area under the concentration-time curve by 19% (geometric mean ratio 0.81, 90% confidence interval [CI] 0.67–0.97), compared to baseline administration of rosuvastatin by itself.[235] Interestingly, however, when giving EGCG for ten days prior to dosing with rosuvastatin, there was no significant AUC reduction compared to baseline. A similar decrease in AUC after acute dosing with atorvastatin and either 300 mg or 600 mg of dried green tea extract is also reported, from an RDBPCT of twelve healthy subjects, though the effect was not dose dependent.[236]

Quite striking decreases in nadolol concentration have also been reported with green tea as a beverage when it was consumed either along with or an hour before nadolol dosing.[237] With concomitant administration, the geometric mean ratio for AUC of nadolol with green tea versus nadolol alone was 0.371 (90% CI 0.303–0.439); with one-hour predosing, the mean ratio was 0.536 (0.406–0.665). Significant reductions in the concentration of lisinopril, given after an overnight fast and concomitantly with 300 mg of EGCG in a water solution, have also been reported, suggesting overall lowered absorption of lisinopril.[238] Further, there have been findings of significant reductions in concentrations of nintedanib with concomitant administration of green tea extract. This effect was most prominent in subjects with a genetic variant of the drug efflux transporter ABCB1 (3435 C>T), a result that suggests alteration of this transporter's activity as a plausible mechanism of action contributing to green tea's effects on pharmacokinetics.[239]

The Ginsengs

Like St. John's wort, *Panax ginseng* appears to increase activity of CYP3A4, as evidenced by lower concentrations of midazolam when the two are concurrently administered in healthy subjects.[240] However, the same work did not show an effect of *Panax ginseng* on inducing p-glycoprotein activity. Highlighting the need for specific human data to clarify drug-herb interactions, consider what is observed clinically when *Panax ginseng*, which would be hypothesized to decrease blood levels of the protease inhibitor ritonavir by increasing CYP3A4 activity, is given for two weeks prior to ritonavir administration. Despite the predicted effect, clinically there does not appear to be any observable impact on the pharmacokinetics of ritonavir at the doses studied. [241] Nor in the same study is any interaction seen between *Panax ginseng* and lopinavir, a drug also metabolized by CYP3A4 and formulated with ritonavir to slow lopinavir's metabolism.[242] Concerning the potential for interaction between *Panax ginseng* and warfarin, two weeks of their concurrent use led to increases in INR and PT of ischemic stroke patients compared to baseline, but there was not a significant across-group difference in INR or PT compared to a group that only received warfarin.[243] An additional study in healthy subjects reported an increase in clearance of warfarin with *Panax ginseng* intake but did not find a change in warfarin's pharmacodynamics that would be clinically relevant.[244]

In subjects with stable coronary heart disease and chronic gastritis, two months of supplementation with saponins from *Panax notoginseng* (a species closely related to *Panax ginseng*) enhanced the antiplatelet effects of aspirin, including reduced platelet aggregation. Moreover, the combination of *notoginseng* and aspirin led to stronger inhibition of platelet production of multiple inflammatory cytokines derived from arachidonic acid and improved symptoms of dyspepsia compared to those in the aspirin group alone.[245]

American ginseng (*Panax quinquefolius*), a third species of the genus *Panax*, has been shown to significantly reduce concentrations (AUC) of warfarin after two weeks of use. In this case, there was also a significant decrease in the INR when introducing American ginseng.[246]

Ginkgo biloba

Ginkgo-drug interactions are also described repeatedly in human studies. In an open-label study of fourteen healthy subjects, standardized *Ginkgo biloba* extract led to a significant reduction in absorption of midazolam (AUC and C_{max}) compared to baseline absorption without ginkgo intake.[247] As in other interaction studies, using midazolam as a marker for effect on the broadly acting metabolizing enzyme CYP3A4. The finding of decreased concentration of midazolam is in contrast to the results seen in another human study of ten healthy subjects, where results showed *Ginkgo biloba* extract significantly increased the absorption of midazolam.[248] The reasons for this discrepancy are not entirely clear.

In the first study, researchers included several drugs, such as lopinavir and ritonavir, and implemented a washout period to minimize their effects. The Uchida study also reported that *Ginkgo biloba* use decreased tolbutamide levels, a drug that CYP2C9 metabolizes. Furthermore, in a small study, *Ginkgo biloba* approximately doubled the maximal blood concentration of the calcium channel blocker nifedipine in two out of eight healthy subjects, which caused headaches, dizziness, and hot flashes in these individuals.[249] Ginkgo administration increased the hydroxylation of omeprazole through the CYP2C19 enzyme, thereby decreasing the blood concentrations of omeprazole in eighteen healthy subjects. Additionally, ginkgo seemed to decelerate the renal clearance of the study's hydroxylated omeprazole form.[250] Interestingly, ginkgo also seemed to slow renal clearance of this study's hydroxylated form of omeprazole.

Echinacea

Another herb with literature available describing its interactions with drugs in vivo is *Echinacea purpurea*. Echinacea leads to an increase in the bioavailability of orally administered midazolam (with differing effects on CYP3A4 activity in the gut and liver), increases blood concentration of orally administered tolbutamide (indicating inhibition of CYP2C9 in the liver), and slows the rate of clearance of orally administered caffeine along with delaying the time to its maximal concentration (indicating inhibition of CYP1A2).[251] The differing effects of echinacea on CYP3A4 in the gut (inhibition) and liver (activation) mean that the effects of echinacea on drugs metabolized by CYP3A4 are probably difficult to predict.

There is also some evidence that echinacea causes small decreases in concentrations of the anti-HIV protease inhibitor darunavir. The change was not substantial enough to merit a change in darunavir dosing, although monitoring darunavir levels during echinacea use is probably warranted.[252] This again illustrates that there is sometimes a gap between establishing a pharmacokinetic interaction and the actual observable impact on drug effect. Finally, one study showed that echinacea can lower plasma levels of warfarin by increasing clearance. However, the observed change in warfarin level did not lead to an actual change in INR; neither was there a change observed in platelet aggregation.[253]

Dong Quai

Sometimes clinicians can observe a probable interaction even when the underlying mechanism of action remains unknown. Several case reports have documented an interaction between warfarin and dong quai. For instance, after taking dong quai for a month, a patient who had been on warfarin for ten years due to a mitral valve replacement experienced widespread bruising and an international normalized ratio (INR) of 10.[254] Similarly, a woman who was taking warfarin to manage her atrial fibrillation observed her prothrombin time and INR more than double after adding dong quai to her regimen for a month. These levels returned to normal once she discontinued the herb.[255]

In sum, there is growing awareness of the interactions between herbs often commonly used in the diet and drugs. Because basic science research may have limited predictive power as to the clinical relevance of an interaction, regularly reviewing the still relatively small but increasing collection of human studies and case reports that document herb-drug interactions in humans is highly important, as is clinical monitoring of patients using both herbal medicines and drugs. We hope that as more is known about how herbs and drugs interact in the body, as our gaps in knowledge are filled, both sets of medicines will become more evenly regarded and utilized.

CHAPTER 10

Drug Interactions with Food and Medicinal Plant Groups

Whether a source of medicinal chemicals is synthetic or natural, everything we take into our body as food, herbs, or drugs has important chemistry that interacts with our biology.

In the previous chapter, we emphasized the need to look at human data as the most definitive and informative evidence to understand interactions between herbs and drugs. However, it is also helpful to identify categories of foods and medicinal plants with shared phytochemistry that may lead to patterns of drug interactions. Rather than approach such associations as definitive contraindications (some of these are common and popular foods), we argue that knowledge of these connections may increase clinicians' awareness of the need to monitor treatment pharmacokinetics and pharmacodynamics.

Here we review findings for the following phytochemicals that may cause drug interactions in groups of foods/herbs: glycoalkaloids from foods in the Solanaceae family; berberine found in barberry and various other herbs; naringin and hesperidin as flavonoids found in citrus; furanocoumarins also found in citrus and medicinal herbs; and sulforaphane and dietary indoles derived from Brassicaceae plants.

Glycoalkaloids from Solanaceae

The nightshade plants from the family Solanaceae (potatoes, tomatoes, eggplant, and peppers) are a dietary source of glycoalkaloids, including solanine and chaconine, the major alkaloids present in potato;[256,257]

hydroxytomatine/tomatine, the major alkaloids in tomato;[258] and solmargine/solasonine, from eggplant.[259] Researchers have also reported the presence of glycoalkaloids in green and red peppers (*Capsicum annuum*),[260] though information as to which specific species of glycoalkaloids are present and predominant is more scarce at present.

Researchers have not shown solanine to have much effect on the drug-metabolizing enzymes of the CYP450 system.[261] However, there are potential interactions between Solanaceae alkaloids and cholinesterase inhibitors that may prove to be clinically relevant. In an in vitro testing system, a concentration of about 34 ppm of chaconine and solanine led to roughly a 25% inhibition of cholinesterase; tomatine also caused inhibition, though at a lower level of about 4%.[262] In vitro studies have also shown that eggplant, particularly aqueous extracts of its peel and pulp, inhibits cholinesterase.[263] In vitro work shows that the cholinesterase-inhibiting effects of solanine and chaconine are more pronounced on butyrylcholinesterase (BuChE) than acetylcholinesterase; moreover, these inhibitory effects on the former enzyme occur with alkaloid concentrations in the nanomolar range, [264] a level that overlaps serum levels obtained after humans eat a serving of mashed potatoes.[265,266]

Further data from McGehee (2019) show that the cholinesterase-inhibitory effects of chaconine and solanine are additive to cholinesterase-inhibiting drugs. Additionally, researchers have demonstrated that chaconine and solanine lead to increased levels of mivacurium (which undergoes metabolism by BuChE) and prolonged mivacurium-induced paralysis in rabbits. Given half-lives for solanine and chaconine of eleven and nineteen hours, respectively, (Hellenas 1992) and some cholinesterase inhibition reported across members of the Solanaceae family, it seems wise to at least be aware of the pattern of consumption of Solanaceae foods before the administration of medications affected by cholinesterase.

Berberine-Containing Herbs

Retailers in the United States now sell berberine as an isolated and purified dietary ingredient. In purified form, this known chemical inhibits multiple drug-metabolizing CYP enzymes, including CYP2D6, CYP2C9, and CYP3A4.[267] Barberry (*Berberis*) and many other plants are known to contain berberine, with some of the fruit being edible and consumed, for example, in Iran.[268] In addition to its occurrence in Berberis species,[269,270] berberine is a recurring attraction also in the Mahonia genus,[271] including *Mahonia aquifolium*, or Oregon grape, popular in jelly and jam recipes for gardeners.[272] In addition, berberine is a constituent of several herbs that may be well-known to many practitioners, goldenseal root,[273] the rhizome of *Coptis chinensis* (Chinese goldthread),[274] as well as several medicinal herbs that may be lesser known, including *Thalictrum foliolosum* (Leafy Meadow-Rue)[275] and *Coscinium fenestratum* (yellow vine).[276]

Flavonoid and Furanocoumarin Drug Interactions

In the previous chapter, we discussed the interactions of green tea's catechins (flavanols within the flavonoid family) with certain medications. Specifically, when given with green tea or its catechins, the concentrations of rosuvastatin,[277] atorvastatin,[278] lisinopril,[279] nadolol,[280] and nintedanib[281] decreased. Naringin, a flavonoid found in grapefruit (which, like other citrus fruits, belongs to the Rutaceae family), was previously suggested as the cause for the inhibition of CYP enzyme activity and the well-documented drug interactions with grapefruit juice.[282] Notably, naringin can elevate felodipine concentrations, a pharmacokinetic change recognized as a reliable indicator of strong CYP3A4 inhibition.[283]

However, while it is true that naringin may act as a competitive inhibitor of CYP3A4 (and relatively high concentrations of naringin exist in fruit segments as compared to juice), it now seems that several furanocoumarin species (Bergamottin, 6'-7-dihydroxybergamottin) are the potent "mechanism-based" irreversible inhibitors of CYP3A4 inhibitors in grapefruit juice.[284] Indeed, grapefruit juice without furanocoumarins yet with flavonoids does not influence the pharmacokinetics of felodipine, which intestinal CYP3A4 processes.[285] Nor, for that matter, has isolated naringin delivered in water at a concentration equivalent to that of juice shown any significant effect on felodipine pharmacokinetics compared to water itself.[286]

Flavonoids also influence drug absorption by affecting the action of a family of membrane transporters called organic anion-transporting polypeptides (OATP). These transporters play a key role in the intestinal absorption of drugs. For example, members of this polypeptide family play a critical role in the uptake of fexofenadine,[287] a common antihistamine, as well as other drugs.[288] Naringin (from grapefruit) and hesperidin (from oranges) each show inhibition of some members of the OATP family in vitro, which would reduce intestinal uptake of drugs moved through this transporter system. In human subjects, grapefruit, orange, and apple juices all significantly reduce the plasma area under the concentration-time curve of fexofenadine.[289] Mechanistically, the uptake of fexofenadine appears to be regulated by the 1A2 polypeptide of the OATP family, with naringin inhibiting OATP1A2 uptake and hesperidin considered likely to mediate the same effect, based on in vitro testing.[290] While furanocoumarins do not seem to impact the uptake of fexofenadine mediated by OATP1A2 (Bailey 2007), there are other members of this polypeptide family inhibited by furanocoumarins in vitro, including potent inhibition of rat OATP3 and OATP1 by 6'-7'-dihydroxybergamottin (Dresser 2002).

Thus, there may be situations where the observed pharmacokinetics of a given drug manifest based on a complex interplay between flavonoids and furanocoumarins affecting both multiple drug transporters and CYP family enzymes (Dresser 2002).

Before concluding our discussion of furanocoumarins, it is also important to note that these important CYP3A4 inhibitors occur not only in grapefruit but also in related fruits, including pomelos (and indeed, pomelos have been shown to alter cyclosporine levels in humans[291]), citrons, and papedas; however, mandarins have virtually no furano-coumarins.[292] Furanocoumarins (bergamottin, 5-methoxypsoralen) have also been reported in bergamot.[293] Thus, where concerns about grapefruit juice and drug interactions exist, the related citrus of concern above should also be avoided, while mandarins may provide a welcome alternative.

Additionally, quite recent work shows aqueous extracts of some plants from both the Apiaceae and Rutaceae families, most notably *Ammi majus* (Queen Anne's lace), *Angelica archangelica* (Norwegian angelica), *Cnidium monnieri* (Monnier's snow parsley), and *Ruta graveolens* (garden rue), are of concern for inhibiting CYP1A2 enzyme function due to furanocoumarin content. Scientists prepared hot water extracts made from gram quantities of these herbs (4.5 g and 9.0 g used to make *A. archangelica* root extracts studied; 6.0 g and 12.0 g used to make *A. majus* seed extracts studied; and 3.0 g used to make *C. monnieri* fruit and R. *graveolens* leaf extracts studied). The furanocoumarins reportedly identified in these extracts (8-methoxypsoralen, 5-methoxypsoralen, and isopsoralen) suggest a slightly different furanocoumarin profile than reported for grapefruit (bergamottin and 6'-7'-dihydroxybergamottin). However, the extracts share the presence of one of the furanocoumarins found in bergamot (5-methoxypsoralen) to date.

Consumption of the herbal extracts led to quite significant differences in caffeine AUC observed in human subjects, with increases ranging between 1.3- and 4.3-fold.[294] A significantly slower clearance of caffeine accompanied these large increases in AUC. Moreover, the authors of this study point to irreversible inhibition of CYP1A2 by the furanocoumarins present (indicated by inhibition being dependent on preincubation time and concentration) and highlight the possibility that binding of the furanocoumarins present in these extracts may lead to the destruction of CYP1A2, thus delaying caffeine metabolism until the body can synthesize new enzyme.

In a highly caffeinated world, ensuring patients know to avoid caffeine when taking extracts from the above species seems especially important. Interestingly, however, grapefruit has not been shown to alter caffeine pharmacokinetics,[295] implying that the difference in furanocoumarin profile between grapefruit and the herbal extracts above leads to functional differences. Whether bergamot might affect caffeine metabolism appears to be unknown at present.

Sulforaphane and Dietary Indoles

Plants from the Brassicaceae family (including cabbage, brussels sprouts, broccoli, cauliflower, radish, turnip, swede, rocket salad, mustard, and wasabi) are the major dietary sources of glucosinolates (sulfur-containing glycosides) in the diet.[296] The enzyme myrosinase hydrolyzes the glucosinolates in many of these vegetables (activated when plant tissue is torn), liberating isothiocyanate compounds, including sulforaphane, deriving from the glucosinolate glucoraphanin. In many of its most commonly consumed food sources, we derive sulforaphane in larger quantities from broccoli, followed by purple cabbage, followed by green cabbage.[297] The indole glucosinolate, glucobrassicin, is broken down by an enzyme, myrosinase, when plant tissue is torn or otherwise broken, forming indole-3-carbinol (I3C).[298] I3C can then polymerize into its dimer, 3,3'-diindolylmethane, as well as other polymers.[299] Both sulforaphane and indole-3-carbinol (and its polymers, collectively referred to here as dietary indoles) may have important effects on drug metabolism, which we briefly discuss below.

Based on in vitro work in Caco-2 cells,[300] there is the potential for sulforaphane to affect the rate of drug metabolism based on changes in the expression of Phase II enzymes such as NADPH: quinine reductase and isoenzymes of glutathione transferase, as well as expression of the gene encoding the cellular drug transporter, multidrug resistance protein. The in vitro data thus far suggest that interactions between sulforaphane and drugs (using furosemide, verapamil, and ketoprofen in the cited study by Lubelska) are very dependent upon the concentration and timing of cellular exposure to both sulforaphane and any given drug. It is thus likely that only in vivo human studies will be able to clarify interactions that exist under usual conditions of use, so human studies exploring sulforaphane-drug interactions are needed. Interestingly, sulforaphane and apigenin, a flavonoid found in sources such as parsley, celery, chamomile, artichokes, and oregano,[301] appear to exert an up to twelvefold increase in the expression of mRNA for the Phase II enzyme UDP-glucuronosyltransferase (1A1), again in a Caco-2 model.[302]

Dietary indoles are unique in that they both induce the activity of CYP enzymes (especially CYP1A1) and inhibit the catalytic activity of the flavin-containing monooxygenase 1 protein, which is also active in drug metabolism. In vitro work using a rat liver microsome model suggests the potential for altered toxicity for drugs, such as tamoxifen and nicotine, that undergo metabolism via both enzyme pathways.[303] Also, dietary indoles have demonstrated inhibitory activity on the drug efflux transporter p-glycoprotein, both in vitro and in mice. Here again, work in humans is needed to understand the composite effects of dietary indoles on drug metabolism.

Like other areas of drug interaction data, human data can best clarify which interactions are of clinical concern. However, thinking about shared chemistry in foods and herbs may increase clinical awareness of potential interactions with drugs and foster appropriate monitoring. This approach also fosters the recognition of foods and herbs as sources of chemistry with equal relevance—natural contributors to health care—highlighting their significant role alongside pharmaceuticals in comprehensive treatment strategies.

CHAPTER 11

Exploring Decentralized Clinical Trials

We began our book by carefully examining the most common scientific tool used to collect data that inform decisions about what we take into our bodies as medicine. As we approach the concluding chapters of this book, we return to the topic of research, pointing forward to how the best data can be gathered in the future. We think that in the rapidly changing world we live in, real-world data such as can be obtained in decentralized clinical trials and observation studies done with the scale of national databases is going to shape our future decision-making in profound ways. In this chapter we take some time to examine one of the most critical instruments for future gathering of real-world data, the decentralized clinical trial (DCT).

Not surprisingly, we commonly think of clinical trials as being conducted in clinics. There are several benefits for the researcher in this traditional approach, including having a central location that handles all subject screening and evaluation consistently, thus limiting variation. However, there are also reasons to embrace a decentralized approach to clinical trials, where at least some or even all of the activities associated with the trial do not occur at a traditional clinical site. Chief among these is the convenience of the patient, a factor that impacts recruitment and retention, as we explore below. As we contemplate the increasing incidence of DCTs, a compelling question emerges as to how the shift in control away from institutions and researchers to patients, who will increasingly participate in a location of their choosing and collect much of the data themselves using provided equipment, may impact the amount of data obtained, as well as its cost and quality.

As we broach the terminology associated with this topic, we also wonder if the useful and broad term of DCT might be complemented (or even replaced) by other terms that more specifically describe how the information in a given DCT is collected. A term such as "entirely remote trial," or ERT, might be a more informative descriptor for a trial conducting all its data collection online and remotely. In contrast, "partially remote trial," or PRT, might be helpful to describe a trial that collects some data through remote participation and other data through a clinical site or multiple clinical sites. This chapter primarily explores the potential of decentralized clinical trials in which all trial activities are managed remotely and online.

DCTs and Subject Recruitment and Retention

One significant obstacle in the traditional clinical trial model is the lack of availability of suitable trials in the local area of eligible patients who are willing and able to take part. For example, an estimate from 2019 suggests that about half or more of patients with cancer (55.6%, CI 43.7–67.3%) do not have a clinical trial available to them at the institution where they receive treatment.[304] In addition to a lack of geographically available clinical trials, subjects still must overcome transportation obstacles to even relatively nearby trials, sacrifice their time, and deal with the weight of risks associated with study intervention, all when they are often not feeling well.

These and other obstacles make the collection of clinical trial data arduous and explain why so many trials fail to recruit to their target level or even terminate due to lack of recruitment and/or retention. An estimate indicates that in the NLM's clinical trial repository, 19% of the registered Phase 2 and Phase 3 clinical trials marked as closed in 2011 were either completed with less than 85% of their target population or terminated early due to recruitment challenges.[305] For a longer-term perspective on this issue, we also point to data from 2006 to 2015 showing that over that time period, 11% of over 13,700 cardiovascular studies were terminated, with the leading cause (41% of the time) being termination from lack of recruitment.[306] Thus it's not uncommon for inadequate subject recruitment to either limit the data available for analysis or to prevent the data collected from being fully useful. Nor is it uncommon for inadequate subject recruitment to either preclude the data ultimately available for analysis or limit the gathering of data to its most useful degree. This situation is problematic both for researchers seeking to answer vital questions and for subjects who participate in studies at various risk levels only to find their efforts have limited usefulness. These issues in recruitment and retention present an ethical dilemma: is it fair to ask subjects to accept study risks, conveying the belief that their participation will lead to meaningful results, even when there is a substantial chance that their involvement may not produce usable data?

For further context on recruitment and retention challenges, it is perhaps useful to step back and consider the related issue of the overall low level of participation from the pool of potentially eligible subjects. One study estimates that only about 5% of eligible subjects choose to participate in clinical trials.[307] Thus we are making inferences about the effect of an intervention after not examining its impact in 95% of a relevant population where many individual differences in response to a drug occur. In some cases, perhaps this sampling and other structuring of the research are adequate to lead to reasonably accurate inferences of what to expect in a population. But perhaps in other circumstances it is not, such as when there is any impactful amount of self-selection bias present. Given the amount of contradictory evidence that emerges when there is an effort to replicate clinical trial results,[308] some reservation about the overall strength of the current level of sampling seems warranted. Surely, obtaining larger and more informative samples through DCTs, as compared to traditional clinical trials, should be welcome news to the research community.

Relatedly, the sample of subjects recruited for most clinical studies used to generate FDA approval of an intervention may not be representative of national demographics and thus may not provide insight into effects like pharmacogenetic impacts that vary by race. For example, worldwide trials, including US-based and internationally based trials, used for FDA approval of drugs and biologics between 2015 and 2019 included Black or African Americans as 7% of study subjects,[309] while the US 2020 census indicates that Black or African Americans constitute 13.6% of the population.[310] Interestingly, it appears that trials done for the sake of approval specifically within the United States are much better at representing Black or African American subjects than internationally based trials, with Black or African Americans representing 16% of study subjects in the United States,[311] perhaps reflecting domestic implementation of FDA guidance encouraging racial diversity in trial recruitment.[312] However, only 2% of study subjects in internationally based trials are Black or African American.

Conversely, where the rate of participation of Asian subjects is concerned, this population is underrepresented in US-centered trials (constituting 2% of US trial subjects[313] whereas Asians constitute 6.3% of the U.S population).[314] Yet when considering the impact of internationally based trials on overall participant demographics, we find that Asians represent 11% of total study subjects enrolled in worldwide trials used for FDA approval. It is certainly the case that some studies done for the purpose of drug approval need to be purposely designed with a higher ratio of a racial group in mind, based on higher prevalence within a certain group. For example, studies of sickle cell anemia will need to recruit a higher percentage of black subjects than white. However, the above data illustrates the complex problem and work that needs to be done to achieve and maintain appropriate rates of racial inclusion in domestic and international trials of drugs destined for the general population.

Can decentralized clinical trials significantly help to increase recruitment and retention of subjects representing the diversity of the national population while not being undermined by unacceptable variability and poor precision? The full answer to that is yet to be known, but some interesting initial learnings appear in the literature.

A first learning is that subjects seem to like participating in clinical trials online. In an analysis of three remote trials with 706 subjects, researchers found that 97% of subjects reported overall satisfaction with the experience of their trial participation being through internet visits.[315] Moreover, when researchers offer remote trial subjects a choice of participation via telephone or through interaction via an internet portal, subjects overwhelmingly choose participation through the internet portal. For example, in the ADAPTABLE trial, where this choice was offered, 13,172 subjects opted for participation through the internet portal compared to 1,904 opting for participation via telephone calls through the call center.[316]

A rare silver lining to the COVID pandemic is the stimulation of researchers to explore decentralized clinical trials to collect data. Estimates are that the recruitment rate into clinical trials decreased by about 74% comparing May 2020 to May 2019.[317] Naturally, researchers began exploring other avenues for getting work done. One of the more interesting studies published during this period is the DeTAP trial, a single-arm observational study of one hundred subjects with atrial fibrillation who were recruited, screened, enrolled, and assessed completely remotely.[318] This study demonstrates "pandemic-proof recruitment and engagement," an apt description given its results.

Two weeks into the study, the research team introduced recruitment through social media ads. Direct outreach had recruited six subjects, but the team found social media recruitment far more effective, attracting ninety-four subjects in twelve days with several hundred on a waitlist. The six-month study demonstrated high compliance: 91% of subjects completed their study televisits, 85% finished their surveys, and 90%

accurately reported blood pressure and 6-lead ECG data using the provided instruments. The subjects submitted this data through a study-specific app. Additionally, over 80% of the participants expressed willingness to continue in clinical research poststudy. However, the demographic makeup of the study—90% White, 3% Black, 4% Asian, and primarily urban residents—highlights the need to focus recruitment in DCTs to underrepresented groups. Possible features of such outreach might be social media ads written with cultural sensitivity to underrepresented racial groups and, where needed, written in the first language of potential subjects.

The DeTAP trial is not alone in finding that subjects strongly prefer participation in research through a decentralized approach. Though smaller in size, a recent study by Sommer[319] found that an option for participation through teleconsultation for screening and telemedicine visits (a decentralized arm) led to enrollment of eighteen subjects, whereas recruitment via health clinics into an arm requiring an on-site visit enrolled only five subjects. Moreover, the recruitment through the decentralized approach successfully recruited from ten of the Swiss cantons (territorial units within Switzerland) and within a rural environment, while the conventional arm recruited from only two cantons. This bodes well for the potential of DCTs with wide-enough reach in advertising to recruit diversely not only with regard to geography but also other demographics, such as economic status.

An additional study of patients with atopic dermatitis from Denmark that required eligible subjects to return a DNA sample prior to enrollment identified 164 potential subjects in eleven days of online recruitment. From the initial group of potential subjects, sixty-five individuals met all the inclusion criteria and were asked to provide a DNA sample before enrollment, a task completed by fifty-five subjects. Of these fifty-five enrolled subjects, fifty-three completed the study, for a retention rate of 96%. This suggests that even with some logistical back-and-forth with eligible subjects before enrollment, it is still possible to recruit and retain subjects efficiently within the structure of a DCT.

How Does the Use of a Decentralized Approach Impact the Observation Effect?

In addition to overcoming obstacles that lead to poor recruitment and retention, decentralized clinical trials allow the researcher to collect a form of real-world data with potentially broad applicability. As we have explored in previous chapters, one of the drawbacks of traditional clinical trials is that they produce data with internal but not necessarily external validity. The results describe what happened in the group studied, but the ability to translate those results to the real world is limited. Perhaps contributing to this conundrum is a phenomenon common to both quantum physics and clinical trials: the observation effect. The presence of an observation effect means that the results of an experiment are affected by the act of watching. In the case of patients, they behave differently when they are aware that they are participating in a clinical trial. Comment on this issue explains that an observation effect in clinical trial research is specifically called the Hawthorne effect and that similar to the effect in quantum physics, a greater intensity of observation over time will lead to a greater observation effect.[320]

At this point, we don't know how much the observation effect impacts data collected in the real world when subjects actively collect data themselves and forward it to researchers instead of data being collected by researchers at a clinical site. However, there is at least a happy possibility that subjects in a space of their choosing will feel less observed and thus have less propensity to change their behavior. Such a decrease in observation effect could, in turn, offset some increase in variability that may occur when research activities are removed from a more tightly controlled clinical site. For right now, what seems safe is to simply recognize that the relatively new approach to clinical research represented by DCTs, with data ascertained in the less-controlled environment of the real world, will collect data with different variability than a more traditional, centralized clinical trial,[321] likely due to a combination of factors. Moreover, if there are some changes in variability of the data collected but the data obtained have greater applicability and can be obtained more easily, on the whole we may look back in some years and be satisfied with the change in course.

Closing Thoughts

As well as unknowns, there are exciting possibilities associated with the promulgation of decentralized clinical trials. While the impacts of subjects collecting data outside of a highly controlled clinical environment are yet to be fully understood, DCTs present an opportunity for data collection that is more convenient, and thus more inviting, to potential subjects. Online recruitment through tools such as social media ads, which might increase participation in trials generally,[322] allows for subjects to be obtained across greater geographical areas and may be tailored to facilitate participation from portions of the population underrepresented in clinical trials. There are indications at this early stage that subject retention in DCTs may also be quite strong and that many subjects are satisfied with their participation in DCTs. Further, DCTs allow for data to be collected within the real-world circumstances of a subject's life.

In addition to the possible benefits above, we should recognize that fast-moving factors are shaping the world of clinical research. While we have highlighted the COVID pandemic as the most recent, conspicuous example, it is probably not the last event to make clinical research that relies heavily on on-site clinical visits more difficult. Moreover, although on-site visits are the only responsible or practical method for collecting certain data, other data can be effectively collected by sending devices or surveys directly to subjects and encouraging them to return results. A research paradigm that continues to rely rigidly or nearly exclusively on on-site data collection for information that can be reasonably collected remotely is unnecessarily vulnerable to interruption. Using a decentralized approach wherever possible not only meets the desire of the subject for more convenient participation; it also allows research to continue even when on-site research centers must close for a time.

On the whole, despite the unknowns inherent in transitioning to a decentralized approach, it seems that now is a moment of opportunity to embrace and facilitate the advent of decentralized clinical research. Doing so paves the way for a health care landscape more informed by real-world data representative of health care consumers.

CHAPTER 12

Understanding Health Basics in the Face of the Unknown

Up to this point, we have covered a great deal of science in order to understand how drugs and herbal medicines are researched, work in our bodies, and interact with each other and foods. Our purpose is to help researchers find truth and to help both patients and practitioners use drugs, herbs, and foods in more informed, efficacious, and safe ways. Our goal is to make medicine whole. Perhaps no such effort by a naturopathic doctor and an herbalist could be complete without sharing important principles that can be applied to maintain good health, which is the concise focus of this last chapter.

In the introduction, we emphasized that despite all the incredible advancements in medical knowledge, we still have a lot to learn about the structure and function of the human body. The first example we gave was the recent discovery, through updated microscopic analysis of frozen tissue, of what may be the largest organ in the body, the interstitium. This isn't the only example of recent basic structure and function discoveries. Experts have taught us about the three layers of meningeal tissue surrounding the brain for many years. It turns out that there is a fourth layer that is very important for allowing the movement of solutes between cerebrospinal fluid and venous blood while also contributing to immune function.[323] Also related to the brain, medicine once believed that functional cells of the brain (neurons) could not regenerate. While this may be true for some areas of brain tissue, there are now at least two areas of the adult brain known to grow new neurons,[324] showing that the brain's structure is more dynamic than previously thought.

Beyond refinements in knowledge of our structure, our understanding of how the body functions may well undergo fundamental shifts in the next generation or two. Clinicians deal with people's bodies and organs on a very macroscopic, often tactile level. Thus it is not surprising that the full application of quantum mechanics to the practice of medicine is a bit of a tough sell (though MRI machines make use of these principles already). Quantum mechanics describe how particles move and interact in a way that the physics of Isaac Newton cannot describe. This is the complex inner world where particles can behave as waves, waves can behave as particles, particles can exist in simultaneous places, and particles that are linked together can continue to behave as connected even when separated by large distances.

It is enough to make the head swim, and it is no wonder physicians with sick people to care for haven't had much time to think about it. But just as aspects of quantum mechanics end up being the only way we can explain how a robin can follow the magnetic fields of the earth (Earth's magnetic field influences the possible states of spin in pairs of free radicals made inside the bird's retina, allowing the robin to detect the earth's magnetic field[325,326]), as the tools of medicine look into ever-tinier spaces in the body, it may well be that some of our greatest advances come by understanding how principles of quantum mechanics govern physiology; this is the emerging field of quantum biology.[327] Perhaps someday, medicine will be more about restoring the correct combination of particle spin in and around cells than dusting a particular receptor with pharmacotherapy.

So if we are anticipating a future in which a lot of our current understanding ends up looking quite crude, is there a rack upon which we can hang our coats of current choices for health preservation that will still matter? There is. While understanding of biology and medicine will continue to change and progress, some principles of good health have already stood the test of time. These include a healthy diet and removing toxic substances from the body wherever possible. We need to take in clean fuel, and we need to effectively take out the cellular trash.

Combined with reasonable exercise and restful sleep, these cornerstones of health will continue to be relevant for as long as people are concerned about maximizing their health. What follows are some of the most succinct guidelines you could hope for in the area, as there is power in simplicity.

Basics of a Healthy Diet

The body can turn just about any source of digestible carbohydrate, fat, and protein into energy. Essentially, this flexibility in metabolic input is like having three different kinds of fuel tanks attached to a unique converter that transforms all the various inputs into a standard fuel burned by the engine. This means that whether you are an Eskimo surviving off marine game or a farmer in India sitting down to a dinner of eggplant and rice, your body will be able to take in the fuel and make energy to keep your processes going. That said, over time some inputs lead to better outcomes in health than others.

To grasp what constitutes a nutritious diet, looking at the broader dietary pattern rather than isolating specific healthy or unhealthy foods is critical. Analyzing overall eating patterns reveals that a diet rich in whole grains, fruits, vegetables, legumes, nuts, unsaturated vegetable oils, and fish, along with choices of lean meat or poultry when meat is included, aligns with a lower risk of mortality from all causes. Conversely, diets that frequently include red and processed meats, high-fat dairy products, and refined carbohydrates or sweets are linked to a higher risk of death from all causes.[328]

If you need more specific motivation to make changes, consider this: one way to help induce heart disease in a mouse model (admittedly in mice who are already genetically predisposed to heart disease) is to give them a diet that is relatively high in both saturated fat and sugar.[329] That is, researchers who want to understand heart disease in humans find it very useful to combine these two components in high amounts for the purpose of inducing heart disease in a predisposed animal.

In humans, while the data on saturated fat intake may sometimes be contradictory, a recent analysis including data from over one million subjects concluded that diets high in saturated fat intake are associated with higher rates of death from all causes, as well as from cardiovascular disease and cancer in particular. Any time a specific set of data gets to the point that it includes information from over a million subjects, it is probably informative to pay attention. On the other hand, the same analysis shows that diets high in polyunsaturated fat (found in plants) are associated with a lower risk of death from all causes and from cardiovascular disease and cancer specifically.[330] So it is better to eat more plants than animals. With regard to sugar, total sugar intake is also associated with an increased risk of death from all causes, as well as from cardiovascular disease in particular.[331]

There are a lot of interesting nuances and specific nutritional topics to explore in the scientific literature (you can spend many years in this area and never become bored), and qualified health-care practitioners can provide well-informed, personalized advice to patients, taking into account individual differences and aiming to achieve specific goals.

In whatever case, though, we should be very cautious about advice that takes us too far away from the overall healthy pattern for too long.

Taking out the Trash

The body is incredible and, frankly, intelligent. It takes in the elements from our environment that we need to function, separates what we need, and gets rid of most of what we don't through rather elegant processes of biotransformation and elimination. A whole book, or several, could be written on supporting these processes, and there are a lot of differing opinions on what is most beneficial. Here we will focus on the evidence for one basic approach, fasting, followed by insight from Dr. Bramwell's past practice as a naturopathic physician, where he used simple hydrotherapy tools to help the body cleanse itself.

Fasting

An excellent review on this topic points out that fasting is a trait shared not only by mammals but also by more simple organisms.[332] Fasting causes many adaptive changes in the cell that reduce oxidative damage and inflammation, enhance energy metabolism, and improve cellular protection.[333] In fact, with regard to the newer discovery of neurogenesis in select areas of the brain, which we mentioned earlier, there is some evidence that caloric restriction can enhance the development of these new brain cells. In us humans, fasting is also a deeply ingrained behavior that, as pointed out in several of the previous citations, is something that Muslims, Christians, Jews, Buddhists, Hindus, and other religious groups agree is important. That ought to tell us something. From this perspective, the practice of fasting may have been with us for as long as, or even longer than, herbal medicine.

Yet there is still a great deal to know about the effects of different forms of fasting, with research now being spurred by the growing interest in intermittent fasting (often eating during a period of six hours during the day and fasting the other eighteen).[334] We do know that some longer forms of fasting, which really must be done under medical supervision, such as eight-day water-only fasts, can be an effective treatment of hypertension.[335] As this area of research starts to develop more fully, one simple approach that may provide benefit is to consistently respect and reinforce our normal, daily physiological period of fasting by strictly stopping eating after a 5:00 p.m. or 6:00 p.m. evening meal until breakfast the next morning and then punctuating that daily pattern with a monthly whole-day fast. Of course, if you have diabetes or other diseases that would be adversely affected by fasting, you need to work with your physician before even doing that. A conversation about fasting might be good for them too.

Hydrotherapy

The roots of using water medicine run deep in naturopathic medicine, tracing back to the use of water applications by Sebastian Kneipp.[336] The essential idea of hydrotherapy is that applications of water of various temperatures can stimulate the body's healing by inducing a hormetic response. As an example of this: while staying in cold water too long will lead to hypothermia, exposure to regulated amounts of cold water stimulates circulation to an area, enhancing the body's ability to increase the number of white blood cells[337] and thus deal with infectious microbes. Indeed, responding to an application of cold water over a site of infection in the respiratory tract may stimulate the body to increase circulation to the area, resulting in greater activity of immune-fighting cells such as neutrophils. While trials on the approach are still few, most naturopathic physicians with experience in practice using hydrotherapy to treat infections, and inflammation generally, would tell you this is an invaluable modality.

An example of one of naturopathic medicine's favorite hydrotherapy treatments is "hot sock / cold sock" to treat nasal congestion. Before bed, the feet are placed in a warm foot bath. After that pleasant experience, the feet are dried and a pair of thin socks soaked in cold water (first wrung out well!) are placed on the feet and then covered with a second pair of dry socks (often wool is preferred for the outer pair of dry socks). This cold stimulation to the feet causes a reflexive reaction of increased blood flow in the head, as has been measured in the nasal mucosa.[338] Many a child with a middle ear infection has awoken the day after such a treatment with marked pain relief. While some will still need antibiotic and/or analgesic treatment, and thus monitoring with a physician is very necessary, this simple intervention could prevent many prescriptions. One of the best pieces of evidence Dr. Bramwell ever saw in support of this treatment was when his then three-year-old daughter was found on the bathroom counter next to the sink getting her cold socks ready. She had a sniffle and knew what to do. If we taught our children to first use hydrotherapy for self-care when appropriate, the world might be quite different!

Another wonderful, though initially uncomfortable, treatment is to put on a thin T-shirt wet with cold water (again wrung out well) and then cover that with a sweatshirt before going to bed (again, please work with a knowledgeable physician because the shock of the cold may not be something that people with conditions like asthma or coronary heart disease can tolerate). Many a mild upper respiratory infection has retreated due to this intervention.

These are just some of the simplest approaches long practiced by naturopathic physicians to help the body clean itself. The interventions are inexpensive and helpful, and often the physicians prescribing them find themselves less and less needed by patients who grow in their capacity to care for their basic health needs. Combined with a consistent pattern of healthy diet as outlined above, reasonable exercise, restful sleep, and the informed and judicious use of the right herbal medicine at the right time, these simple interventions really can improve the health of many and lead to more sparing use of pharmacotherapy.

Closing Thoughts on Informed Health Freedom

After reading this book, you hopefully see a place for the informed, wise use of herbal medicines and other dietary supplements. In order to ensure that you have access to these medicines and unfiltered information as to how they may best be used, we'll close with some important thoughts on maintaining, and indeed expanding, health freedom.

For many years, US media has maintained a steady drumbeat: dietary supplements (including herbal remedies) are unregulated, unsafe, and ineffective. Nothing could be further from the truth. Heavy regulation is imposed on supplements, and with relatively rare exceptions, they are safer than pharmaceutical drugs when used prudently. They are also remarkably effective when used correctly. One author of this book has experience providing patient care in an outpatient environment, using both supplements and pharmaceutical drugs—though favoring minimal use of the latter—to cater to the daily health needs of patients. Another author owns a dietary supplement business and frequently receives appreciation from customers who notice a positive impact on their health from the supplements. The truth is, the right supplement at the right time for the right person makes a real difference.

Supplements are generally food-based medicine that is simply different than pharmaceutical medicine. Supplements rightfully, and after considerable upheaval, now have a distinct regulatory structure that reflects the fact that they are more food-based. As observed below, when FDA primarily views drug companies as its main clients, it can sometimes lead to decisions that have costly consequences paid with human lives. Furthermore, an FDA perspective that perceives the supplement industry as a lesser priority or even as a challenge can potentially restrict valuable information about natural disease-treating options that consumers should have available to them.

First, FDA sees the pharmaceutical industry, rather than the American public, as its client. This reality came into focus in light of the tragedy of Vioxx, when FDA ignored its experts' warning about safety to get Vioxx to market, resulting in up to 60,000 deaths of Americans due to heart attacks. In response to this tragedy, landmark congressional testimony was given by Dr. David Graham, who worked at FDA for twenty-three years. Dr. Graham summed things up concisely when he stated the following, referring to FDA's Center for Drug Evaluation and Research (CDER), which approves new drugs [our text added to quotation]:

> CDER's culture regards industry as the agency's primary client rather than as an entity in need of regulation. The agency's bias toward drug approval, noted by the IOM [Institute of Medicine], is enshrined in PDUFA [the Prescription Fee Act that enables FDA to charge drug companies to review their data prior to approval], which requires FDA to negotiate with industry over how user fees shall be spent. Patients and consumers, the public, get no seat at the table.[339]

While FDA does need to assess drug applications efficiently, it currently obtains almost half (46%) of its total $6.2 billion operating budget and fees from drug companies, and these fees account for 66% of the Human Drug Program budget.[340] While charging drug companies fees to assess the data they provide does help the drug review process become more efficient, it also promotes proindustry bias and increases drug costs, which are then passed on to users. Moreover, the rate of drugs entering the market that later need a market withdrawal or black box warning due to postapproval discovery of serious toxicity has not decreased since FDA started charging user fees, and may have gone up. As we have described, before 1992, the rate of these actions was estimated to be 21.2%. However, by 2014, this rate reportedly increased to 26.7%. This change in rate occurred after the introduction of user fees in 1992.[341] If we put more money into the drug-approval system but increase the rate at which dangerous products are allowed, we have a process that is seriously flawed.

In contrast, FDA does not gain financially from the regulation of the dietary supplement industry. In fact, for many years, FDA has wanted to control and limit public access to supplements, or at least control what is said about supplements, as the agency does with pharmaceutical drugs. In the late 1980s and early 1990s, in a series of actions known as the black currant oil cases,[342] FDA attacked supplements as unapproved food additives. In the course of these actions, the agency deemed it necessary to conduct an armed raid on a doctor's office where licensed and trained clinicians were merely administering vitamin and mineral injections to their patients.[343] Most would agree that bulletproof vests are a bit of an extreme reaction to such clinical care.

Americans were outraged, producing the biggest letter-writing campaign to Congress since the Vietnam War[344] and driving the Dietary Supplement Health and Education Act (DSHEA) of 1994. In the thirty years since DSHEA, the supplement industry has grown exponentially, from around four billion dollars then[345] to over sixty billion dollars now.[346] Consumers have more, better, and cheaper supplements and health information than ever before. FDA argues that all this growth requires more regulation. On the contrary, it clearly shows that free markets work and that Americans don't need FDA to make their own informed choices. It also shows that free markets, like the republic, work best when citizens tell the government what to do, not the reverse. DSHEA is based on the liberty principle (allowed unless harmful), while FDA still clings to PMA (premarket approval, or "illegal unless allowed"), a New Deal era way of thinking.

Under DSHEA, dietary supplements aren't drugs, so they can't be used to diagnose, treat, cure, or prevent diseases, no matter how much historical, scientific, or popular support they may have. Currently, only FDA can approve drugs to treat diseases. FDA views pharmaceutical companies, not the public, as its client. It takes a dim view of traditional medicine, and very few herbal-based medicines are approved for disease treatment. At the time of this writing, this includes two botanical drugs available for prescription use, as well as some herbal substances such as psyllium that are available in over-the-counter drugs.[347] The dietary supplement category now includes many herbal ingredients and formulas that were long thought of as drugs and effectively used to diagnose, treat, cure, or prevent disease, as well as to maintain good health. Regulations should be altered so that herbal medicines can communicate both their traditionally recognized and newly discovered therapeutic values. Many medicinal plants still exist but may need to be grown commercially again. Innovators should have a regulatory space that allows them to create new herbal medicines or craft formulas from ancient recipes, and explain their effects accurately without FDA declaring these herbal medicines to be "unapproved new drugs."

While FDA requires clinical trials to approve new drugs, DSHEA does not require clinical trials for supplements, and indeed the cost of new clinical trials for every supplement would make them as expensive as pharmaceuticals. Most supplement companies base their claims (such as they are allowed by law to make) on published ingredient research by third-party researchers—much as this book has done. This is consistent with both the letter and spirit of DSHEA, which was intended to keep regulation to a bare minimum, in a free market.

However, FDA is not the only government agency that regulates what is communicated about the effects of supplements, and to provide a full picture of the current danger to dietary supplements, it is important to highlight recent actions of the Federal Trade Commission, or FTC. In March 2023, FTC sent a "Notice of Penalty Offenses" letter to nearly 700 supplement companies warning them that any claim they make without substantiation that FTC considers adequate could incur financial penalties of over $50,000 per violation.[348,349] One problem with FTC's blanket Notice of Offense letter was that it did not highlight a single specific claim of concern that would let companies know what kind of statement was currently the focus of the commission's thinking. This unsubstantiated warning of possibly unsubstantiated claims isn't very helpful.

A bigger problem, however, is FTC's emphasis on replicated findings from clinical trials as a basis for adequate substantiation.[350] While replication of results sounds wonderful and would be ideal, the practical truth is that replication in clinical trials can be elusive and some even say we are living in a "replication crisis," in part because we simply cannot assume that different study populations will respond to studied medicines in the same way.[351] It is not unusual for even highly respected, oft-cited clinical trials to have results that are contradictory with other trials in the same body of evidence.[352]

Especially when it comes to substantiation for today's nondisease claims, we need to be aware of regulatory creep by both FDA and FTC and remember what DSHEA actually says about substantiation, which is simply that to make a claim the manufacturer of a dietary supplement needs to have "substantiation that said statement is truthful and not misleading."[353] There is not a legal definition of what exactly constitutes substantiation. Moreover, we need to always bear in mind the stated intent of Congress in passing DSHEA, which is that "the Federal government should not take any actions to impose unreasonable regulatory barriers limiting or slowing the flow of safe products and accurate information to consumers."[354] Don't slow the flow. It would be tragic for FTC to repeat the same mistakes of overreach committed by FDA that precipitated the need for passage of DSHEA.

This does not mean that FTC does not have important work to do. The commission should go after fraud when someone claims to cure serious diseases without some reasonable basis of evidence. But if fraud defines one end of the substantiation spectrum, then enforceable criteria for adequate substantiation created by a government agency that doesn't understand the importance of both clinical trial data and empirical evidence in traditional medicines define the other. Each claim has a unique body of evidence that should be examined by those with expertise in the field, expertise that FTC does not have. A claim should not be precluded if experts in the industry can provide reasonable assurance that the claim is truthful, based on both historical evidence and a body of evidence that continues to evolve over time.

Rather than taking upon itself the role of "changing the dynamics of the marketplace," as FTC wrote in the Notice of Penalty Offenses letter (not appropriate in a free market system), FTC could better utilize its talents to work with and rely upon qualified industry experts to ensure that evidence reasonably supports claims industry makes. For example, while it's fair to require that a claim to be able to treat a disease have evidence from human research, it should also be fair for a company to say that an ingredient has been traditionally used to treat a disease if that statement can be defended historically.

There also should be room for supplements to claim disease treatment when credible data support such a claim. Current law allows only FDA-approved drugs to treat disease, regardless of evidence. Because FDA (and FTC if they overstep their role) determines available drug options and claims, the agency acts as a de facto monopoly, limiting what Americans can choose and why. Every monopoly (government or otherwise) limits supply and competition, driving high prices and windfall profits and injuring consumers both through high prices and in the consumers' avoidance of treatment. In addition, many consumers (and providers) cannot understand the risks of the approved drugs because toxicity curves are not fully defined before drug approval. When this shortcoming is combined with the reality that potential options or accurate and full information about options are disallowed, patients are not well served and medicine is not whole.

Consumers need safe, effective, and affordable choices, and to date, regulation hasn't delivered. Responsible suppliers in a free market can provide good options, as they have shown under DSHEA. Ultimately, effective and affordable products are best judged by customers, not regulators. Moreover, products that don't meet a real customer need at an affordable price won't last long in a competitive market. Finally, while FTC can prevent some fraud, in a competitive, transparent market, private litigants play an even more important and defining role as they seek available remedy in law.

In short, the many dysfunctions of our current drug system are often the unintended result of well-intended but misguided or imbalanced regulation. We should encourage truthful discourse, responsible innovation, and new kinds of scientific inquiry and evidence. Informed choice, healthy competition, free markets, and transparency are often better solutions than one-size-fits-all regulation and enforcement with its many unintended consequences.

We hope that this book has been both interesting and informative and that it will encourage more thought and conversations about the benefits and science of herbal medicine, both traditional and modern. We believe these benefits include:

- A wide and varied toolbox to address individual needs
- An earlier, safer, gentler approach to maintaining good health
- Ingredients and medicines that are more affordable, sustainable, and biodegradable
- No monopoly or oligopoly to artificially limit options or inflate prices
- Regional and local sourcing, reducing transportation and addressing local needs

In addition, herbal medicine has long embraced complex formulation, which offers many advantages over the conventional "one disease, one target, one drug" (magic bullet) model, including:

- Lower doses that reduce risk of serious adverse events
- More predictable results across individual variations (portfolio effect)
- Better handling of side effects and interactions
- More results from less medicine

Much of the content in this book was previously featured in the *Townsend Letter for Doctors*. We're thankful to our editors there for letting us publish this material in this format. Ultimately, we believe that education paves the way for informed and healthy choices. Please feel free to share your observations and experiences with us too! We all have so much to learn and too little time and experience with which to do it.

May we have the health and wisdom
to help others to health and wisdom!

Afterword

In reading this book, some will undoubtedly think it is a "hit piece" on conventional medicine. After all, we show that the RCT, the so-called "gold standard" of modern pharmacology, is fundamentally flawed in several ways. We dismiss the "magic bullet" model as a simplifying assumption without evidentiary basis. We find that small doses of many ingredients can be empirically effective and clinically preferable, though this may be harder to show with statistical certainty. But these findings don't negate anything in Western medicine. In fact, they are based on Western medicine's own observations, merely viewed a little differently. They prompt us to reconsider the assumption that Western medicine is infallible and question the dismissal of centuries of empirical wisdom from the East. But then, we knew that assumption was wrong already, right? It's like saying the Egyptians weren't architects because they didn't have circular saws or cement mixers.

Thomas Jefferson was by far the most scientific president we've ever had. He served as president of the American Philosophical Society, the nation's oldest scientific body, during his entire term and for many years before and after his presidency. He wrote only one book: his *Notes on the State of Virginia*, written at the height of the Revolutionary War, in part during a forced exile from Monticello. In chapter 17, "On Religion," Jefferson warned of the dangers of mixing politics and government into matters of both science and religion. After reciting the long history of religious oppression in both England and the Colonies, he wrote:

Reason and free enquiry are the only effectual agents against error. Give a loose to them, they will support the true religion, by bringing every false one to their tribunal, to the test of their investigation. They are the natural enemies of error, and of error only. Had not the Roman government permitted free enquiry, Christianity could never have been introduced. Had not free enquiry been indulged, at the aera of the reformation, the corruptions of Christianity could not have been purged away. *If it be restrained now, the present corruptions will be protected, and new ones encouraged. Was the government to prescribe to us our medicine and diet, our bodies would be in such keeping as our souls are now.* Thus in France the emetic was once forbidden as a medicine, and the potato as an article of food. Government is just as infallible too when it fixes systems in physics. Galileo was sent to the inquisition for affirming that the earth was a sphere: the government had declared it to be as flat as a trencher, and Galileo was obliged to abjure his error. This error however at length prevailed, the earth became a globe, and Descartes declared it was whirled round its axis by a vortex. The government in which he lived was wise enough to see that this was no question of civil jurisdiction, or we should all have been involved by authority in vortices. In fact, the vortices have been exploded, and the Newtonian principle of gravitation is now more firmly established, on the basis of reason, than it would be were the government to step in, and to make it an article of necessary faith. Reason and experiment have been indulged, and error has fled before them. *It is error alone which needs the support of government. Truth can stand by itself.* (emphasis added)

What was obvious to Jefferson and others in 1784 is much more obvious today. The government has no business telling doctors (or anyone else) what constitutes valid science or what is "disinformation." Censorship is as wrong today as it ever was. If speech is false or fraudulent, legal avenues exist for recourse. However, in scientific inquiry, the principle of free inquiry must always prevail, with acceptance of the best evidence until superior evidence comes along.

Stating that modern medicine has its flaws or acknowledging the skills of ancient practitioners, despite their limited tools, should not be controversial. As we turn the final page to the beginnings of this thoughtful discussion, let us recognize the immense potential of striving for a health care system that respects the depth of ancient wisdom while advancing through modern science and pursuing a path to more holistic care. An open dialogue among health care professionals, free from the constraints of overregulation and prejudice, is essential for a dynamic exchange of ideas and therapies. The power of advocacy at the individual and community levels cannot be understated; it is crucial for encouraging a system that includes diverse healing methods. Further, our dedication is unshakable: we stand committed to informing, engaging in dialogue, and supporting the campaign for health freedom. With the insights from this volume, we hope to bridge the gap between traditional and contemporary medicine, enriching both fields and ultimately improving patient care.

Acknowledgments

I am indebted to my coauthor Ben, without whom I could not have tackled this project. My parents unwittingly set me on this path some twenty-four years ago; it has been a joyous journey. My siblings kindly let me continue to play in this sandbox after our parents passed, and they make me laugh. My team at RidgeCrest Herbals are inspired and devoted lovers of all things herbal, and I love them for it. My wife Carol has tolerated many nights of me coming to bed late with "square eyeballs" from looking at a computer screen. My three girls and four grandkids keep me younger inside than I look on the outside. Finally, a special thanks to Amanda Dubaić and Nina Matijašević, who kept this project on track from the other side of the world despite busy lives and families of their own. It could not have happened without you!

—MW

I express great appreciation to Matt for the opportunity to research and write this book with him and for the tireless work of Amanda Dubaić and Nina Matijašević to somehow pull everything together. Matt and I have had many thoughtful conversations spawned by our findings in the literature, scientific and historical, that have framed the thoughts, insights, and opinions expressed in this book. An end goal for me is for this work to move forward a thoughtful discussion, more generally, both with those who agree and those who disagree with the perspectives presented. I would also like to thank all the researchers and scientists whose work is cited in this book and those who have moved the science of healing forward from one generation to another as hardworking researchers and clinicians in many fields. There are many healing heroes in medicine. While the purpose of this book, in part, is to help us reexamine our approach to how we define, obtain, and apply evidence in medicine, I have nothing but the greatest respect for any and all who use the best available means to find ways to help restore us to health when we are sick. Thank you. Thanks also to my wife, Nanette, for supportively listening as each part of this book has unfolded.

—BB

Endnotes

1. Benias PC, Wells RG, Sackey-Aboagye B, et al. Structure and distribution of an unrecognized interstitium in human tissues. *Sci Rep* 2018;8:4947. https://doi.org/10.1038/s41598-018-23062-6. See also https://nyulangone.org/news/nyu-school-medicine-pathologist-uncovers-potential-new-organ-setting-fiery-debate. Accessed July 31, 2023. And Stewart RH. A modern view of the interstitial space in health and disease. *Front Vet Sci.* 2020 Nov 5;7:609583. doi: 10.3389/fvets.2020.609583. PMID: 33251275; PMCID: PMC7674635.

2. https://en.wikipedia.org/wiki/Falsifiability. Accessed August 8, 2023.

3. https://www.pbs.org/wgbh/nova/article/falsifiability/. Accessed August 8, 2023.

4. https://www.nbcnews.com/science/cosmic-log/scientists-find-medicinal-plants-caught-neanderthal-teeth-flna894410. Accessed July 31, 2023.

5. Halberstein RA. Medicinal plants: historical and cross-cultural usage patterns. *Ann Epidemiol.* 2005 Oct;15(9):686–699. doi: 10.1016/j.annepidem.2005.02.004. PMID: 15921929.

6. Cardiac valvulopathy associated with exposure to fenfluramine or dexfenfluramine: U.S. Department of Health and Human Services interim public health recommendations, November 1997. *MMWR.* 1997 November 14;46(45):1061–1066.

7. https://lfsblaw.com/fen-phen-diet-drug-lawsuit/. Accessed July 31, 2023.

8. Budnitz DS, Shehab N, Lovegrove MC, Geller AI, Lind JN, Pollock DA. US emergency department visits attributed to medication harms, 2017–2019. *JAMA*. 2021 Oct 5;326(13):1299–1309. doi: 10.1001/jama.2021.13844. PMID: 34609453; PMCID: PMC8493432.

9. Gøtzsche PC. Our prescription drugs kill us in large numbers. *Pol Arch Med Wewn*. 2014;124(11):628–634. doi: 10.20452/pamw.2503. Epub 2014 Oct 30. PMID: 25355584.

10. https://www.who.int/initiatives/medication-without-harm.

11. Light DW, Lexchin J, Darrow JJ. Institutional corruption of pharmaceuticals and the myth of safe and effective drugs (June 1, 2013). *Journal of Law, Medicine and Ethics*. 2013;14(3):590–610, Available at SSRN: https://ssrn.com/abstract=2282014.

12. https://ethics.harvard.edu/blog/new-prescription-drugs-major-health-risk-few-offsetting-advantages.

13. Tabish SA. Complementary and alternative healthcare: Is it evidence-based? *Int J Health Sci* (Qassim). 2008 Jan;2(1):V–IX. PMID: 21475465; PMCID: PMC3068720.

14. https://hbr.org/2019/01/the-art-of-evidence-based-medicine.

15. Severus E, Laber E, Lipkovich I. Double-blind randomized placebo-controlled trials in the treatment of affective disorders: problems and alternatives. *Current Treatment Options Psychiatry*. 2015; 2(3):262–270.

16. Neppe, VN. Limitations of the double-blind pharmaceutical study. http://www.pni.org/psychopharmacology/doubleblind/ DoubleBlindNeppe.pdf. Accessed August 1, 2023.

17. Bonaccio M, Di Castelnuovo A, Costanzo S, Persichillo M, De Curtis A, Cerletti C, Donati MB, de Gaetano G, Iacoviello L; Moli-sani Study Investigators. Interaction between Mediterranean diet and statins on mortality risk in patients with cardiovascular disease: findings from the Moli-sani Study. *Int J Cardiol*. 2019 Feb 1;276:248-254. doi: 10.1016/j.ijcard.2018.11.117. Epub 2018 Nov 24. PMID: 30527993.

18. Collier R. Legumes, lemons and streptomycin: a short history of the clinical trial. *CMAJ*. 2009 Jan 6;180(1):23–24. doi: 10.1503/cmaj.081879. PMID: 19124783; PMCID: PMC2612069.

19. Haygarth J. Of the imagination as a cause and cure of disorders of the body, exemplified by fictitious tractors. *Ann Med* (Edinb). 1800;5:133–145. PMCID: PMC5111928.

20. Stolberg M. Inventing the randomized double-blind trial: the Nuremberg salt test of 1835. *J R Soc Med*. 2006 Dec;99(12):642–643. doi: 10.1177/014107680609901216. PMID: 17139070; PMCID: PMC1676327.

21. Clarke M. The 1944 patulin trial of the British Medical Research Council. J R Soc Med. 2006 Sep;99(9):478-80. doi: 10.1177/014107680609900923. PMID: 16946394; PMCID: PMC1557884.

22. MRC Streptomycin in Tuberculosis Trials Committee. Streptomycin treatment of pulmonary tuberculosis. *BMJ*. 1948;ii:769–783. See also Crofton J. The MRC randomized trial of streptomycin and its legacy: a view from the clinical front line. *J R Soc Med*. 2006 Oct;99(10):531–534. doi: 10.1177/014107680609901017. PMID: 17021304; PMCID: PMC1592068.

23. Public Law 87-781-October 10, 1962. Drug Amendments of 1962. https://www.govinfo.gov/content/pkg/STATUTE-76/pdf/STATUTE-76-Pg780.pdf. Accessed September 22, 2023.

24. Temin P. *Taking Your Medicine: Drug Regulation in the United States*. Harvard University Press; 1980:126–127.

25. National Research Council. *Drug Efficacy Study: Final Report to the Commissioner of Food and Drugs—Food and Drug Administration*. The National Academies Press;1969. https://doi.org/10.17226/24615.

26. 34 FR 14596-14597. September 19, 1969. https://archives.federalregister.gov/issue_slice/1969/9/19/14595-14600.pdf#page=5. Accessed September 22, 2023.

27. Demonstrating substantial evidence of effectiveness for human drug and biological products: guidance for industry. U.S. Department of Health and Human Services Food and Drug Administration Center for Biologics Evaluation and Research (CBER) Center for Drug Evaluation and Research (CDER) December 2019.

28. https://www.accessdata.fda.gov/scripts/cdrh/cfdocs/cfcfr/cfrsearch.cfm?fr=314.126. Accessed September 27, 2023.

29. Junod, SW. FDA and clinical drug trials: a short history. U.S. Food & Drug Administration. Accessed September 22, 2023. https://www.fda.gov/media/110437/download#:~:text=several%20kinds%20of%20randomized%20controlled,been%20referred%20to%20as%20the%20%22. Originally published as "FDA and clinical drug trials: a short history," in *A Quick Guide to Clinical Trials, Madhu Davies and Faiz Kerimani*, eds. Bioplan Inc.; 2008:25–55.

30. Downing NS, Aminawung JA, Shah ND, Krumholz HM, Ross JS. Clinical trial evidence supporting FDA approval of novel therapeutic agents, 2005–2012. *JAMA*. 2014 Jan 22–29;311(4):368–377. doi: 10.1001/jama.2013.282034. PMID: 24449315; PMCID: PMC4144867.

31. Fisher RA. *The Design of Experiments*. Reprint of the 8th edition. Hafner Publishing Company, Inc. (reprinted by arrangement);1971:19.

32. Saint-Mont U. Randomization does not help much, comparability does. *PLoS One*. 2015 Jul 20;10(7):e0132102. doi: 10.1371/journal.pone.0132102. PMID: 26193621; PMCID: PMC4507867.

33. Nguyen T-L, Collins GS, Lamy A, Devereaux PJ, Daurès JP, Landais P, Le Manach Y. Simple randomization did not protect against bias in smaller trials. *Journal of Clinical Epidemiology*.

34. Senn S. Empirical studies of balance do not justify a requirement for 1,000 patients per trial. *J Clin Epidemiol*. 2022 Aug;148:184–188. doi: 10.1016/j.jclinepi.2022.02.010. Epub 2022 Mar 4. PMID: 35248697.

35. Nguyen TL, Xie L. Incomparability of treatment groups is often blindly ignored in randomized controlled trials—a post hoc analysis of baseline characteristic tables. *J Clin Epidemiol*. 2021 Feb;130:161–168. doi: 10.1016/j.jclinepi.2020.10.012. Epub 2020 Oct 17. PMID: 33080343.

36. Hróbjartsson A, Forfang E, Haahr MT, Als-Nielsen B, Brorson S. Blinded trials taken to the test: an analysis of randomized clinical trials that report tests for the success of blinding. *Int J Epidemiol*. 2007 Jun;36(3):654–663. doi: 10.1093/ije/dym020. Epub 2007 Apr 17. PMID: 17440024.

37. Feinstein AR. Clinical biostatistics. IX. How do we measure "safety and efficacy"? *Clin Pharmacol Ther*. 1971 May–Jun;12(3):544–558. doi: 10.1002/cpt1971123544. PMID: 5567805.

38. Meldrum, ML. "Departures from the design": the randomized clinical trial in historical context, 1946–1970. Dissertation for Doctor of Philosophy in History. State University of New York at Stony Brook. December 1994.

39. Richard Carter. *Breakthrough: The Saga of Jonas Salk*. Trident Press;1966:170–171.

40. Meldrum M. "A calculated risk": the Salk polio vaccine field trials of 1954. *BMJ*. 1998 Oct 31;317(7167):1233–1236. doi: 10.1136/bmj.317.7167.1233. PMID: 9794869; PMCID: PMC1114166.

41. Richard Carter. *Breakthrough: The Saga of Jonas Salk*. Trident Press;1966:190–193.

42. Francis T. Evaluation of the 1954 poliomyelitis vaccine field trial: further studies of results determining the effectiveness of poliomyelitis vaccine (Salk) in preventing paralytic poliomyelitis. *J Am Med Assoc*. 1955 Aug 6;158(14):1266–1270. doi: 10.1001/jama.1955.02960140028004. PMID: 14392076.

43. Gup T, Neumann J. Experimental drugs: death in the search for cures. *Washington Post*. October 18, 1981.

44. National Cancer Institute's Therapy Program, Joint Hearing before the Subcommittee on Health and the Environment of the Committee on Energy and Commerce (House of Representatives) and the Subcommittee on Investigations and Oversight of the Committee on Science and Technology, 97th Congress, 1st Session, October 27, 1981. U.S. Government Printing Office; 1981. 154. See also Rothman DJ, Edgar H. Scientific rigor and medical realities: placebo trials in medical research. In: Fee E, Fox DM, eds. *AIDS: The Making of a Chronic Disease*. University of California Press;1992:194–206.

45. https://www.cancer.gov/about-cancer/treatment/clinical-trials/what-are-trials/placebo Accessed September 26, 2023.

46. Anglemyer A, Horvath HT, Bero L. Healthcare outcomes assessed with observational study designs compared with those assessed in randomized trials. *Cochrane Database Syst Rev*. 2014 Apr 29;2014(4):MR000034. doi: 10.1002/14651858.MR000034.pub2. PMID: 24782322; PMCID: PMC8191367.

47. Concato J, Shah N, Horwitz RI. Randomized, controlled trials, observational studies, and the hierarchy of research designs. *N Engl J Med*. 2000 Jun 22;342(25):1887–1892. doi: 10.1056/NEJM200006223422507. PMID: 10861325; PMCID: PMC1557642.

48. Resnik DB. Beyond post-marketing research and MedWatch: long-term studies of drug risks. *Drug Des Devel Ther*. 2007;1:1–5. doi:10.2147/dddt.s2352

49. DAD Study Group, Friis-Møller N, Reiss P, Sabin CA, Weber R, Monforte Ad, El-Sadr W, Thiébaut R, De Wit S, Kirk O, Fontas E, Law MG, Phillips A, Lundgren JD. Class of antiretroviral drugs and the risk of myocardial infarction. *N Engl J Med*. 2007 Apr 26;356(17):1723–1735. doi: 10.1056/NEJMoa062744. PMID: 17460226.

50. Gilmartin-Thomas JF, Liew D, Hopper I. Observational studies and their utility for practice. *Aust Prescr*. 2018 Jun;41(3):82–85. doi: 10.18773/austprescr.2018.017. Epub 2018 Jun 1. PMID: 29922003; PMCID: PMC6003013.

51. Demonstrating substantial evidence of effectiveness with one adequate and well-controlled clinical investigation and confirmatory evidence: guidance for industry. U.S. Department of Health and Human Services Food and Drug Administration Oncology Center of Excellence (OCE) Center for Biologics Evaluation and Research (CBER) Center for Drug Evaluation and Research (CDER) September 2023.

52. Ioannidis JP. Why most published research findings are false. *PLoS Med*. 2005 Aug;2(8):e124. doi: 10.1371/journal.pmed.0020124. Epub 2005 Aug 30. Erratum in: *PLoS Med*. 2022 Aug 25;19(8):e1004085. PMID: 16060722; PMCID: PMC1182327.

53. Budnitz DS, Shehab N, Lovegrove MC, Geller AI, Lind JN, Pollock DA. US emergency department visits attributed to medication harms, 2017–2019. *JAMA*. 2021 Oct 5;326(13):1299–1309. doi: 10.1001/jama.2021.13844. PMID: 34609453; PMCID: PMC8493432.

54. https://www.census.gov/popclock/. Accessed April 4, 2023.

55. Solomon DH, Husni ME, Libby PA, Yeomans ND, Lincoff AM, Lüscher TF, Menon V, Brennan DM, Wisniewski LM, Nissen SE, Borer JS. The risk of major NSAID toxicity with celecoxib, ibuprofen, or naproxen: a secondary analysis of the PRECISION trial. *Am J Med*. 2017 Dec;130(12):1415–1422.e4. doi: 10.1016/j.amjmed.2017.06.028. Epub 2017 Jul 26. PMID: 28756267.

56. Obeid S, Libby P, Husni E, Wang Q, Wisniewski LM, Davey DA, Wolski KE, Xia F, Bao W, Walker C, Ruschitzka F, Nissen SE, Lüscher TF. Cardiorenal risk of celecoxib compared with naproxen or ibuprofen in arthritis patients: insights from the PRECISION trial. *Eur Heart J Cardiovasc Pharmacother*. 2022 Sep 3;8(6):611–621. doi: 10.1093/ehjcvp/pvac015. PMID: 35234840.

57. Bavry AA, Thomas F, Allison M, Johnson KC, Howard BV, Hlatky M, Manson JE, Limacher MC. Nonsteroidal anti-inflammatory drugs and cardiovascular outcomes in women: results from the women's health initiative. *Circ Cardiovasc Qual Outcomes*. 2014 Jul;7(4):603–610. doi: 10.1161/CIRCOUTCOMES.113.000800. Epub 2014 Jul 8. PMID: 25006185; PMCID: PMC4151243.

58. Collins AJ, Davies J, Dixon SA. Contrasting presentation and findings between patients with rheumatic complaints taking nonsteroidal anti-inflammatory drugs and a general population referred for endoscopy. *Br J Rheumatol*. 1986 Feb;25(1):50–53. doi: 10.1093/rheumatology/25.1.50. PMID: 3484649.

59. Shah AA, Thjodleifsson B, Murray FE, Kay E, Barry M, Sigthorsson G, Gudjonsson H, Oddsson E, Price AB, Fitzgerald DJ, Bjarnason I. Selective inhibition of COX-2 in humans is associated with less gastrointestinal injury: a comparison of nimesulide and naproxen. *Gut*. 2001 Mar;48(3):339–346. doi: 10.1136/gut.48.3.339. PMID: 11171823; PMCID: PMC1760142.

60. Maiden L, Thjodleifsson B, Seigal A, Bjarnason II, Scott D, Birgisson S, Bjarnason I. Long-term effects of nonsteroidal anti-inflammatory drugs and cyclooxygenase-2 selective agents on the small bowel: a cross-sectional capsule enteroscopy study. *Clin Gastroenterol Hepatol*. 2007 Sep;5(9):1040–1045. doi: 10.1016/j.cgh.2007.04.031. Epub 2007 Jul 10. PMID: 17625980.

61. Laine L, Curtis SP, Langman M, Jensen DM, Cryer B, Kaur A, Cannon CP. Lower gastrointestinal events in a double-blind trial of the cyclo-oxygenase-2 selective inhibitor etoricoxib and the traditional nonsteroidal anti-inflammatory drug diclofenac. *Gastroenterology*. 2008 Nov;135(5):1517–1525. doi: 10.1053/j.gastro.2008.07.067. Epub 2008 Aug 3. PMID: 18823986.

62. Washio E, Esaki M, Maehata Y, Miyazaki M, Kobayashi H, Ishikawa H, Kitazono T, Matsumoto T. Proton pump inhibitors increase incidence of nonsteroidal anti-inflammatory drug-induced small bowel injury: a randomized, placebo-controlled trial. *Clin Gastroenterol Hepatol*. 2016 Jun;14(6):809–815.e1. doi: 10.1016/j.cgh.2015.10.022. Epub 2015 Oct 30. PMID: 26538205.

63. Moris G, Garcia-Monco JC. The challenge of drug-induced aseptic meningitis. *Arch Intern Med*. 1999 Jun 14;159(11):1185–1194. doi: 10.1001/archinte.159.11.1185. PMID: 10371226.

64. For a useful tool that compares how the concentration of morphine equivalents varies among different prescribed opioid drugs, see https://www.oregonpainguidance.org/opioidmedcalculator/.

65. Banta-Green CJ, Merrill JO, Doyle SR, Boudreau DM, Calsyn DA. Opioid use behaviors, mental health and pain—development of a typology of chronic pain patients. *Drug Alcohol Depend*. 2009 Sep 1;104(1–2):34–42. doi: 10.1016/j.drugalcdep.2009.03.021. Epub 2009 May 26. PMID: 19473786; PMCID: PMC2716214.

66. Boscarino JA, Rukstalis M, Hoffman SN, Han JJ, Erlich PM, Gerhard GS, Stewart WF. Risk factors for drug dependence among out-patients on opioid therapy in a large US health-care system. *Addiction*. 2010 Oct;105(10):1776–1782. doi: 10.1111/j.1360-0443.2010.03052.x. Epub 2010 Aug 16. PMID: 20712819.

67. Young RA, Fulda KG, Espinoza A, Gurses AP, Hendrix ZN, Kenny T, Xiao Y. Ambulatory medication safety in primary care: a systematic review. *J Am Board Fam Med*. 2022 May–Jun;35(3):610–628. doi: 10.3122/jabfm.2022.03.210334. PMID: 35641040; PMCID: PMC9730343.

68. Gregory H, Cantley M, Calhoun C, Hall GA, Matuskowitz AJ, Weant KA. Incidence of prescription errors in patients discharged from the emergency department. *Am J Emerg Med*. 2021 Aug;46:266–270. doi: 10.1016/j.ajem.2020.07.061. Epub 2020 Jul 25. PMID: 33046298.

69. Gregory H, Cantley M, Hall GA, Matuskowitz AJ, Weant KA. Incidence of anticoagulation medication prescribing errors in patients discharged from the emergency department. *Journal of the American College of Clinical Pharmacy*. 2020 Nov;3(7):1280–5.

70. Raymond J, Parrein P, Barat E, Chenailler C, Decreau-Gaillon G, Varin R, Joly LM. Pharmacist tracking and correction of medication errors: an improvement project in the observation ward of the emergency department. *Ann Pharm Fr*. 2023 Jun 23:S0003-4509(23)00067-6. doi: 10.1016/j.pharma.2023.06.004. Epub ahead of print. PMID: 37356662.

71. Leili M, Nikvarz N. Evaluating the role of clinical pharmacist in the detection and reduction of medication errors in a specialized burn unit. *Burns*. 2023 May;49(3):646–654. doi: 10.1016/j.burns.2022.04.013. Epub 2022 Apr 22. PMID: 35610074.

72. Naseralallah LM, Hussain TA, Jaam M, Pawluk SA. Impact of pharmacist interventions on medication errors in hospitalized pediatric patients: a systematic review and meta-analysis. *Int J Clin Pharm*. 2020 Aug;42(4):979–994. doi: 10.1007/s11096-020-01034-z. Epub 2020 Apr 24. PMID: 32328958.

73. Hamel C, Tortolano L, Bermudez E, Desmaris R, Klein S, Slimano F, Lemare F. Computerized pediatric oncology prescriptions review by pharmacist: a descriptive analysis and associated risk factors. *Pediatr Blood Cancer*. 2018 Apr;65(4). doi: 10.1002/pbc.26897. Epub 2017 Dec 18. PMID: 29251399.

74. Lim WY, Hss AS, Ng LM, John Jasudass SR, Sararaks S, Vengadasalam P, Hashim L, Praim Singh RK. The impact of a prescription review and prescriber feedback system on prescribing practices in primary care clinics: a cluster randomized trial. *BMC Fam Pract*. 2018 Jul 19;19(1):120. doi: 10.1186/s12875-018-0808-4. PMID: 30025534; PMCID: PMC6053727.

75. Osmani F, Arab-Zozani M, Shahali Z, Lotfi F. Evaluation of the effectiveness of electronic prescription in reducing medical and medical errors (systematic review study). *Ann Pharm Fr*. 2023 May;81(3):433–445. doi: 10.1016/j.pharma.2022.12.002. Epub 2022 Dec 10. PMID: 36513154; PMCID: PMC9737496.

76. Langley JN. On the reaction of cells and of nerve-endings to certain poisons, chiefly as regards the reaction of striated muscle to nicotine and to curari. *J Physiol*. 1905 Dec 30;33(4–5):374–413. doi: 10.1113/jphysiol.1905.sp001128. PMID: 16992819; PMCID: PMC1465797.

77. AHLQUIST RP. A study of the adrenotropic receptors. *Am J Physiol*. 1948 Jun;153(3):586–600. doi: 10.1152/ajplegacy.1948.153.3.586. PMID: 18882199.

78. Abimbola Farinde. Drug receptor interactions. Reviewed June 2021, Modified September 2022. Merck Manual Professional Version.

79. Kenakin T. Receptor theory. *Curr Protoc Pharmacol*. 2008 Jun;Chapter 1:Unit1.2. doi: 10.1002/0471141755.ph0102s41. PMID: 22294216.

80. Caffrey AR, Borrelli EP. The art and science of drug titration. *Ther Adv Drug Saf*. 2021 Jan 19;11:2042098620958910. doi: 10.1177/2042098620958910. PMID: 33796256; PMCID: PMC7967860.

81. Robinson CA, Siu A, Meyers R, Lee BH, Cash J. Standard dose development for medications commonly used in the neonatal intensive care unit. *J Pediatr Pharmacol Ther*. 2014 Apr;19(2):118–126. doi: 10.5863/1551-6776-19.2.118. PMID: 25024672; PMCID: PMC4093664.

82. Chatelut E, White-Koning ML, Mathijssen RH, Puisset F, Baker SD, Sparreboom A. Dose banding as an alternative to body surface area-based dosing of chemotherapeutic agents. *Br J Cancer*. 2012 Sep 25;107(7):1100–1106. doi: 10.1038/bjc.2012.357. Epub 2012 Aug 28. PMID: 22929884; PMCID: PMC3461153.

83. https://www.fda.gov/media/160036/download.

84. Kenakin T. Receptor theory. *Curr Protoc Pharmacol*. 2008 Jun;Chapter 1:Unit1.2. doi: 10.1002/0471141755.ph0102s41. PMID: 22294216.

85. Littleton J. Receptor regulation as a unitary mechanism for drug tolerance and physical dependence—not quite as simple as it seemed! *Addiction*. 2001 Jan;96(1):87–101. doi: 10.1046/j.1360-0443.2001.961877.x. PMID: 11177522.

86. Dubois M, Pickar D, Cohen M, Gadde P, Macnamara TE, Bunney WE. Effects of fentanyl on the response of plasma beta-endorphin immunoreactivity to surgery. *Anesthesiology*. 1982 Dec;57(6):468–472. doi: 10.1097/00000542-198212000-00006. PMID: 6293344.

87. Hargreaves KM, Dionne RA, Mueller GP, Goldstein DS, Dubner R. Naloxone, fentanyl, and diazepam modify plasma beta-endorphin levels during surgery. *Clin Pharmacol Ther*. 1986 Aug;40(2):165–171. doi: 10.1038/clpt.1986.159. PMID: 3731680.

88. Burgos N, Toloza FJK, Singh Ospina NM, Brito JP, Salloum RG, Hassett LC, Maraka S. Clinical outcomes after discontinuation of thyroid hormone replacement: a systematic review and meta-analysis. *Thyroid*. 2021 May;31(5):740–751. doi: 10.1089/thy.2020.0679. Epub 2020 Dec 29. PMID: 33161885; PMCID: PMC8110016.

89. https://powo.science.kew.org/taxon/urn:lsid:ipni.
org:names:30016176-2. Accessed August 21, 2023.

90. Hussain AI, Anwar F, Nigam PS, Ashraf M, Gilani AH. Seasonal variation in content, chemical composition and antimicrobial and cytotoxic activities of essential oils from four Mentha species. *J Sci Food Agric*. 2010 Aug 30;90(11):1827–1836. doi: 10.1002/jsfa.4021. PMID: 20602517.

91. Melguizo-Rodríguez L, García-Recio E, Ruiz C, De Luna-Bertos E, Illescas-Montes R, Costela-Ruiz VJ. Biological properties and therapeutic applications of garlic and its components. *Food Funct*. 2022 Mar 7;13(5):2415–2426. doi: 10.1039/d1fo03180e. PMID: 35174827.

92. https://extension.oregonstate.edu/news/herbs-rescue-fend-deer-aromatic-plants#:~:text=%E2%80%93%20Many%20 of%20the%20plants%20that,animals%20that%20find%20them%20 unpalatable. Accessed August 21, 2023.

93. Ried K, Frank OR, Stocks NP. Aged garlic extract reduces blood pressure in hypertensives: a dose-response trial. *Eur J Clin Nutr*. 2013 Jan;67(1):64–70. doi: 10.1038/ejcn.2012.178. Epub 2012 Nov 21. PMID: 23169470; PMCID: PMC3561616.

94. Hiki N, Kurosaka H, Tatsutomi Y, Shimoyama S, Tsuji E, Kojima J, Shimizu N, Ono H, Hirooka T, Noguchi C, Mafune K, Kaminishi M. Peppermint oil reduces gastric spasm during upper endoscopy: a randomized, double-blind, double-dummy controlled trial. *Gastrointest Endosc*. 2003 Apr;57(4):475–482. doi: 10.1067/mge.2003.156. PMID: 12665756.

95. Abraham Maslow. *The Psychology of Science: A Reconnaissance*. Harper & Row;1966.

96. Grandjean P. Paracelsus revisited: the dose concept in a complex world. *Basic Clin Pharmacol Toxicol*. 2016 Aug;119(2):126–132. doi: 10.1111/bcpt.12622. Epub 2016 Jun 24. PMID: 27214290; PMCID: PMC4942381.

97. Ashauer R, Agatz A, Albert C, Ducrot V, Galic N, et al. Toxicokinetic-toxicodynamic modeling of quantal and graded sublethal endpoints: a brief discussion of concepts. *Environmental Toxicology and Chemistry* 2011;30(11): 2519–2524. ⟨10.1002/etc.639⟩. ⟨hal-01453851⟩.

98. Ledolter J, Abraham B. (1981). Parsimony and its importance in time series forecasting. *Technometrics*, 1981;23(4): 411–414. https://doi.org/10.2307/1268232.

99. Box GEP. Robustness in the strategy of scientific model building. Editors Robert L. Launer, Graham N. Wilkinson. *Robustness in Statistics*. Academic Press;1979:201–236.

100. Gesztelyi R, Zsuga J, Kemeny-Beke A, Varga B, Juhasz B, Tosaki A. The Hill equation and the origin of quantitative pharmacology. *Arch Hist Exact Sci*. 2012;66:427–438.

101. Neubig RR, Spedding M, Kenakin T, Christopoulos A; International Union of Pharmacology Committee on Receptor Nomenclature and Drug Classification. International Union of Pharmacology Committee on Receptor Nomenclature and Drug Classification. XXXVIII. Update on terms and symbols in quantitative pharmacology. *Pharmacol Rev*. 2003 Dec;55(4):597–606. doi: 10.1124/pr.55.4.4. PMID: 14657418.

102. Mercer JM. *Cooperativity: Reference Module in Life Sciences*. Elsevier;2023. ISBN 9780128096338. https://doi.org/10.1016/B978-0-12-822563-9.00093-7.

103. Di Veroli GY, Fornari C, Goldlust I, Mills G, Koh SB, Bramhall JL, Richards FM, Jodrell DI. An automated fitting procedure and software for dose-response curves with multiphasic features. *Sci Rep*. 2015 Oct 1;5:14701. doi: 10.1038/srep14701. PMID: 26424192; PMCID: PMC4589737.

104. https://ehp.niehs.nih.gov/doi/epdf/10.1289/ehp.1003327.

105. https://derangedphysiology.com/main/cicm-primary-exam/required-reading/pharmacodynamics/Chapter%20412/quantal-dose-response-curves. Accessed January 3, 2024.

106. Stanley TH. Anesthesia for the 21st century. *Proc* (Bayl Univ Med Cent). 2000 Jan;13(1):7–10. doi: 10.1080/08998280.2000.11927635. PMID: 16389318; PMCID: PMC1312206.

107. Gilbert-Kawai E, Wittenberg M. Therapeutic index. In *Essential Equations for Anaesthesia: Key Clinical Concepts for the FRCA and EDA*. 79–80. Cambridge University Press;2014. doi:10.1017/CBO9781139565387.040.

108. Gable RS. Comparison of acute lethal toxicity of commonly abused psychoactive substances. *Addiction*. 2004 Jun;99(6):686-696. doi: 10.1111/j.1360-0443.2004.00744.x. PMID: 15139867.

109. Bertolini A, Ferrari A, Ottani A, Guerzoni S, Tacchi R, Leone S. Paracetamol: new vistas of an old drug. *CNS Drug Rev*. 2006 Fall–Winter;12(3-4):250–75. doi: 10.1111/j.1527-3458.2006.00250.x. PMID: 17227290; PMCID: PMC6506194.

110. Gable RS. Comparison of acute lethal toxicity of commonly abused psychoactive substances. *Addiction*. 2004 Jun;99(6):686–696. doi: 10.1111/j.1360-0443.2004.00744.x. PMID: 15139867.

111. https://www.oraulearning.org/topclass/media/a7ab6ff6-ccb2-4f0c-80ca-7a56b7015f8a/02-005.html. Accessed 2023-20-14.

112. Geller AI, Shehab N, Weidle NJ, Lovegrove MC, Wolpert BJ, Timbo BB, Mozersky RP, Budnitz DS. Emergency department visits for adverse events related to dietary supplements. *N Engl J Med*. 2015 Oct 15;373(16):1531–1540. doi: 10.1056/NEJMsa1504267. PMID: 26465986; PMCID: PMC6196363.

113. Budnitz DS, Pollock DA, Weidenbach KN, Mendelsohn AB, Schroeder TJ, Annest JL. National surveillance of emergency department visits for outpatient adverse drug events. *JAMA*. 2006 Oct 18;296(15):1858–1866. doi: 10.1001/jama.296.15.1858. PMID: 17047216.

114. https://www.ncbi.nlm.nih.gov/pmc/articles/PMC5593261. Accessed October 13, 2023.

115. Dimmitt SB, Stampfer HG, Warren JB. The pharmacodynamic and clinical trial evidence for statin dose. *Br J Clin Pharmacol*. 2018 Jun;84(6):1128–1135. doi: 10.1111/bcp.13539. Epub 2018 Apr 16. PMID: 29393975; PMCID: PMC5980555.

116. Dimmitt S, Stampfer H, Martin JH. When less is more—efficacy with less toxicity at the ED50. *Br J Clin Pharmacol*. 2017 Jul;83(7):1365–1368. doi: 10.1111/bcp.13281. Epub 2017 Apr 6. PMID: 28387051; PMCID: PMC5465328.

117. Frank C, Himmelstein DU, Woolhandler S, Bor DH, Wolfe SM, Heymann O, Zallman L, Lasser KE. Era of faster FDA drug approval has also seen increased black-box warnings and market withdrawals. *Health Aff* (Millwood). 2014;33(8):1453–1459.

118. Yang Y, Li X, Chen G, Xian Y, Zhang H, Wu Y, Yang Y, Wu J, Wang C, He S, Wang Z, Wang Y, Wang Z, Liu H, Wang X, Zhang M, Zhang J, Li J, An T, Guan H, Li L, Shang M, Yao C, Han Y, Zhang B, Gao R, Peterson ED; CTS-AMI Investigators. Traditional Chinese medicine compound (Tongxinluo) and clinical outcomes of patients with acute myocardial infarction: the CTS-AMI randomized clinical trial. *JAMA*. 2023 Oct 24;330(16):1534–1545. doi: 10.1001/jama.2023.19524. PMID: 37874574; PMCID: PMC10599127.

119. Tinetti ME, Naik AD, Dodson JA. Moving from disease-centered to patient goals-directed care for patients with multiple chronic conditions: patient value-based care. *JAMA Cardiol*. 2016 Apr 1;1(1):9–10. doi: 10.1001/jamacardio.2015.0248. PMID: 27437646; PMCID: PMC6995667.

120. Calabrese EJ. The emergence of the dose-response concept in biology and medicine. *Int J Mol Sci*. 2016 Dec 5;17(12):2034. doi: 10.3390/ijms17122034. PMID: 27929392; PMCID: PMC5187834.

121. Schulz H, Crump T. NIH-98-134: Contemporary medicine as presented by its practitioners themselves, Leipzig, 1923:217-250. *Nonlinearity Biol Toxicol Med.* 2003 Jul;1(3):295–318. doi: 10.1080/15401420390249880. PMID: 19330137; PMCID: PMC2656124.

122. Calabrese EJ. The emergence of the dose-response concept in biology and medicine. *Int J Mol Sci.* 2016 Dec 5;17(12):2034. doi: 10.3390/ijms17122034. PMID: 27929392; PMCID: PMC5187834.

123. Branham SE. The effects of certain chemical compounds upon the course of gas production by baker's yeast. *J Bacteriol.* 1929 Oct;18(4):247–264. doi: 10.1128/jb.18.4.247-264.1929. PMID: 16559396; PMCID: PMC375082.

124. Hotchkiss M. Studies on Salt Action: VI. The stimulating and inhibitive effect of certain cations upon bacterial growth. *J Bacteriol.* 1923 Mar;8(2):141–162. doi: 10.1128/jb.8.2.141-162.1923. PMID: 16558991; PMCID: PMC379008.

125. Smith EC. Effects of ultra-violet radiation and temperature on fusarium. II. Stimulation. *Bulletin of the Torrey Botanical Club.* 1935; 62(3):151–164.

126. Calabrese EJ, Blain RB. The hormesis database: the occurrence of hormetic dose responses in the toxicological literature. *Regul Toxicol Pharmacol.* 2011 Oct;61(1):73–81. doi: 10.1016/ j.yrtph.2011.06.003. Epub 2011 Jun 15. PMID: 21699952.

127. Calabrese EJ. Hormesis: why it is important to toxicology and toxicologists. *Environ Toxicol Chem.* 2008 Jul;27(7):1451–1474. doi: 10.1897/07-541. PMID: 18275256.

128. Falchetti R, Fuggetta MP, Lanzilli G, Tricarico M, Ravagnan G. Effects of resveratrol on human immune cell function. *Life Sci.* 2001 Nov 21;70(1):81–96. doi: 10.1016/s0024-3205(01)01367-4. PMID: 11764009.

129. Zhang C, Li C, Chen S, Li Z, Ma L, Jia X, Wang K, Bao J, Liang Y, Chen M, Li P, Su H, Lee SM, Liu K, Wan JB, He C. Hormetic effect of panaxatriol saponins confers neuroprotection in PC12 cells and zebrafish through PI3K/AKT/mTOR and AMPK/SIRT1/FOXO3 pathways. *Sci Rep.* 2017 Jan 23;7:41082. doi: 10.1038/srep41082. PMID: 28112228; PMCID: PMC5253660.

130. Bao J, Huang B, Zou L, Chen S, Zhang C, Zhang Y, Chen M, Wan JB, Su H, Wang Y, He C. Hormetic effect of berberine attenuates the anticancer activity of chemotherapeutic agents. *PLoS One.* 2015 Sep 30;10(9):e0139298. doi: 10.1371/journal.pone.0139298. PMID: 26421434; PMCID: PMC4589364.

131. Wang D, Calabrese EJ, Lian B, Lin Z, Calabrese V. Hormesis as a mechanistic approach to understanding herbal treatments in traditional Chinese medicine. *Pharmacol Ther.* 2018 Apr;184:42–50. doi: 10.1016/j.pharmthera.2017.10.013. Epub 2017 Nov 8. PMID: 29080703.

132. Wang D, Calabrese EJ, Lian B, Lin Z, Calabrese V. Hormesis as a mechanistic approach to understanding herbal treatments in traditional Chinese medicine. *Pharmacol Ther.* 2018 Apr;184:42–50. doi: 10.1016/j.pharmthera.2017.10.013. Epub 2017 Nov 8. PMID: 29080703.

133. Paintaud G, Bechtel Y, Brientini MP, Miguet JP, Bechtel PR. Effects of liver diseases on drug metabolism. *Therapie*. 1996 Jul-Aug;51(4):384–389. PMID: 8953814.

134. Talal AH, Venuto CS, Younis I. Assessment of hepatic impairment and implications for pharmacokinetics of substance use treatment. *Clin Pharmacol Drug Dev*. 2017 Mar;6(2):206–212. doi: 10.1002/cpdd.336. PMID: 28263464; PMCID: PMC5859945.

135. Albillos A, de la Hera A, González M, Moya JL, Calleja JL, Monserrat J, Ruiz-del-Arbol L, Alvarez-Mon M. Increased lipopolysaccharide binding protein in cirrhotic patients with marked immune and hemodynamic derangement. *Hepatology*. 2003 Jan;37(1):208–217. doi: 10.1053/jhep.2003.50038. PMID: 12500206.

136. Jover R, Bort R, Gómez-Lechón MJ, Castell JV. Down-regulation of human CYP3A4 by the inflammatory signal interleukin-6: molecular mechanism and transcription factors involved. *FASEB J*. 2002 Nov;16(13):1799–1801. doi: 10.1096/fj.02-0195fje. Epub 2002 Sep 19. PMID: 12354697.

137. Zhuang Y, de Vries DE, Xu Z, Marciniak SJ Jr, Chen D, Leon F, Davis HM, Zhou H. Evaluation of disease-mediated therapeutic protein-drug interactions between an anti-interleukin-6 monoclonal antibody (sirukumab) and cytochrome P450 activities in a phase 1 study in patients with rheumatoid arthritis using a cocktail approach. *J Clin Pharmacol*. 2015 Dec;55(12):1386–1394. doi: 10.1002/jcph.561. Epub 2015 Jul 29. PMID: 26054042.

138. Schmitt C, Kuhn B, Zhang X, Kivitz AJ, Grange S. Disease-drug-drug interaction involving tocilizumab and simvastatin in patients with rheumatoid arthritis. *Clin Pharmacol Ther*. 2011 May;89(5):735–740. doi: 10.1038/clpt.2011.35. Epub 2011 Mar 23. Erratum in: *Clin Pharmacol Ther*. 2011 Sep;90(3):479. Dosage error in article text. PMID: 21430660.

139. Mayo PR, Skeith K, Russell AS, Jamali F. Decreased dromotropic response to verapamil despite pronounced increased drug concentration in rheumatoid arthritis. *Br J Clin Pharmacol*. 2000 Dec;50(6):605–613. doi: 10.1046/j.1365-2125.2000.00314.x. PMID: 11136300; PMCID: PMC2015009.

140. Sanaee F, Clements JD, Waugh AW, Fedorak RN, Lewanczuk R, Jamali F. Drug-disease interaction: Crohn's disease elevates verapamil plasma concentrations but reduces response to the drug proportional to disease activity. *Br J Clin Pharmacol*. 2011 Nov;72(5):787–797. doi: 10.1111/j.1365-2125.2011.04019.x. PMID: 21592185; PMCID: PMC3243013.

141. Stader F, Kinvig H, Penny MA, Battegay M, Siccardi M, Marzolini C. Physiologically based pharmacokinetic modelling to identify pharmacokinetic parameters driving drug exposure changes in the elderly. *Clin Pharmacokinet*. 2020 Mar;59(3):383–401. doi: 10.1007/s40262-019-00822-9. PMID: 31583609.

142. McLean AJ, Le Couteur DG. Aging biology and geriatric clinical pharmacology. *Pharmacol Rev*. 2004 Jun;56(2):163–184. doi: 10.1124/pr.56.2.4. PMID: 15169926.

143. Robertson SS, Mouksassi MS, Varin F. Population pharmaco-kinetic/pharmacodynamic modeling of O-desmethyltramadol in young and elderly healthy volunteers. *Drugs Aging*. 2019 Aug;36(8):747–758. doi: 10.1007/s40266-019-00681-w. PMID: 31161580.

144. Meyers BR, Mendelson MH, Deeter RG, Srulevitch-Chin E, Sarni MT, Hirschman SZ. Pharmacokinetics of cefoperazone in ambulatory elderly volunteers compared with young adults. *Antimicrob Agents Chemother*. 1987 Jun;31(6):925–929. doi: 10.1128/AAC.31.6.925. PMID: 3619425; PMCID: PMC284213.

145. Chu SY, Wilson DS, Guay DR, Craft C. Clarithromycin pharmacokinetics in healthy young and elderly volunteers. *J Clin Pharmacol*. 1992 Nov;32(11):1045–1049. doi: 10.1002/j.1552-4604.1992.tb03809.x. PMID: 1474166.

146. Stader F, Kinvig H, Penny MA, Battegay M, Siccardi M, Marzolini C. Physiologically based pharmacokinetic modelling to identify pharmacokinetic parameters driving drug exposure changes in the elderly. *Clin Pharmacokinet*. 2020 Mar;59(3):383–401. doi: 10.1007/s40262-019-00822-9. PMID: 31583609.

147. Goa KL, Balfour JA, Zuanetti G. Lisinopril: a review of its pharmacology and clinical efficacy in the early management of acute myocardial infarction. *Drugs*. 1996 Oct;52(4):564–588. doi: 10.2165/00003495-199652040-00011. PMID: 8891468.

148. Mishkin GE, Denicoff AM, Best AF, Little RF. Update on enrollment of older adults onto National Cancer Institute national clinical trials network trials. *J Natl Cancer Inst Monogr*. 2022 Dec 15;2022(60):111–116. doi: 10.1093/jncimonographs/lgac017. PMID: 36519819; PMCID: PMC9949562.

149. Veronese N, Petrovic M, Benetos A, Denkinger M, Gudmundsson A, Knol W, Marking C, Soulis G, Maggi S, Cherubini A; a Special Interest Group in Systematic Reviews and Meta-Analyses and the Task Force on Pharmaceutical Strategy of the European Geriatric Medicine Society (EuGMS). Underrepresentation of older adults in clinical trials on COVID-19 vaccines: a systematic review. *Ageing Res Rev*. 2021 Nov;71:101455. doi: 10.1016/j.arr.2021.101455. Epub 2021 Sep 3. PMID: 34487916; PMCID: PMC8413602.

150. Braithwaite HE, Payne T, Duce N, Lim J, McCulloch T, Loadsman J, Leslie K, Webster AC, Gaskell A, Sanders RD. Impact of female sex on anaesthetic awareness, depth, and emergence: a systematic review and meta-analysis. *Br J Anaesth*. 2023 Sep;131(3):510–522. doi: 10.1016/j.bja.2023.06.042. Epub 2023 Jul 14. PMID: 37453840.

151. Storosum BWC, Mattila T, Wohlfarth TD, Gispen-de Wied CC, Roes KCB, den Brink WV, de Haan L, Denys DAJP, Zantvoord JB. Gender differences in the response to antipsychotic medication in patients with schizophrenia: an individual patient data meta-analysis of placebo-controlled studies. *Psychiatry Res*. 2023 Feb;320:114997. doi: 10.1016/j.psychres.2022.114997. Epub 2022 Dec 24. PMID: 36603382.

152. Goldberg AC, Banach M, Catapano AL, Duell PB, Leiter LA, Hanselman JC, Lei L, Mancini GBJ. Evaluation of the efficacy and safety of bempedoic acid in women and men: pooled analyses from phase 3 trials. *Atherosclerosis*. 2023 Nov;384:117192. doi: 10.1016/j.atherosclerosis.2023.117192. Epub 2023 Jul 28. PMID: 37648637.

153. Koonrungsesomboon N, Khatsri R, Wongchompoo P, Teekachunhatean S. The impact of genetic polymorphisms on CYP1A2 activity in humans: a systematic review and meta-analysis. *Pharmacogenomics J*. 2018 Dec;18(6):760–768. doi: 10.1038/s41397-017-0011-3. Epub 2017 Dec 27. PMID: 29282363.

154. White JR Jr, Padowski JM, Zhong Y, Chen G, Luo S, Lazarus P, Layton ME, McPherson S. Pharmacokinetic analysis and comparison of caffeine administered rapidly or slowly in coffee chilled or hot versus chilled energy drink in healthy young adults. *Clin Toxicol* (Phila). 2016;54(4):308–-312. doi: 10.3109/15563650.2016.1146740. PMID: 27100333; PMCID: PMC4898153.

155. Benowitz NL. Clinical pharmacology of caffeine. *Annu Rev Med*. 1990;41:277–288. doi: 10.1146/annurev.me.41.020190.001425. PMID: 2184730.

156. https://www.cdc.gov/diabetes/basics/type2.html. Accessed November 16, 2023.

157. https://www.ncbi.nlm.nih.gov/gene/6580. Accessed November 21, 2023.

158. Singh S, Shukla AK, Usman K, Banerjee M. Pharmacogenetic impact of SLC22A1 gene variant rs628031 (G/A) in newly diagnosed Indian type 2 diabetes patients undergoing metformin monotherapy. *Pharmacogenet Genomics*. 2023 Apr 1;33(3):51–58. doi: 10.1097/FPC.0000000000000493. Epub 2023 Feb 9. PMID: 36853844.

159. Hitman GA, Hawrami K, McCarthy MI, Viswanathan M, Snehalatha C, Ramachandran A, Tuomilehto J, Tuomilehto-Wolf E, Nissinen A, Pedersen O. Insulin receptor substrate-1 gene mutations in NIDDM: implications for the study of polygenic disease. *Diabetologia*. 1995 Apr;38(4):481–486. doi: 10.1007/BF00410287. PMID: 7796990.

160. Clausen JO, Hansen T, Bjørbaek C, Echwald SM, Urhammer SA, Rasmussen S, Andersen CB, Hansen L, Almind K, Winther K, et al. Insulin resistance: interactions between obesity and a common variant of insulin receptor substrate-1. Lancet. 1995 Aug 12;346(8972):397–402. doi: 10.1016/s0140-6736(95)92779-4. PMID: 7623569.

161. Prudente S, Di Paola R, Pezzilli S, Garofolo M, Lamacchia O, Filardi T, Mannino GC, Mercuri L, Alberico F, Scarale MG, Sesti G, Morano S, Penno G, Cignarelli M, Copetti M, Trischitta V. Pharmacogenetics of oral antidiabetes drugs: evidence for diverse signals at the IRS1 locus. *Pharmacogenomics J*. 2018 May 22;18(3):431-435. doi: 10.1038/tpj.2017.32. Epub 2017 Jul 11. PMID: 28696414.

162. Baroni MG, D'Andrea MP, Montali A, Pannitteri G, Barillà F, Campagna F, Mazzei E, Lovari S, Seccareccia F, Campa PP, Ricci G, Pozzilli P, Urbinati G, Arca M. A common mutation of the insulin receptor substrate-1 gene is a risk factor for coronary artery disease. *Arterioscler Thromb Vasc Biol*. 1999 Dec;19(12):2975–2980. doi: 10.1161/01.atv.19.12.2975. PMID: 10591678.

163. https://www.ncbi.nlm.nih.gov/gene/19130. Accessed November 21, 2023.

164. Gong Y, McDonough CW, Beitelshees AL, Karnes JH, O'Connell JR, Turner ST, Chapman AB, Gums JG, Bailey KR, Boerwinkle E, Johnson JA, Cooper-DeHoff RM. PROX1 gene variant is associated with fasting glucose change after antihypertensive treatment. *Pharmacotherapy*. 2014 Feb;34(2):123–130. doi: 10.1002/phar.1355. Epub 2013 Oct 9. PMID: 24122840; PMCID: PMC3945213.

165. Klen J, Dolžan V, Janež A. CYP2C9, KCNJ11 and ABCC8 polymorphisms and the response to sulphonylurea treatment in type 2 diabetes patients. *Eur J Clin Pharmacol*. 2014 Apr;70(4):421–428. doi: 10.1007/s00228-014-1641-x. Epub 2014 Jan 18. PMID: 24442125.

166. Riley J, Ross JR, Rutter D, Wells AU, Goller K, du Bois R, Welsh K. No pain relief from morphine? Individual variation in sensitivity to morphine and the need to switch to an alternative opioid in cancer patients. *Support Care Cancer*. 2006 Jan;14(1):56–64. doi: 10.1007/s00520-005-0843-2. Epub 2005 Jun 11. PMID: 15952009.

167. Bond C, LaForge KS, Tian M, Melia D, Zhang S, Borg L, Gong J, Schluger J, Strong JA, Leal SM, Tischfield JA, Kreek MJ, Yu L. Single-nucleotide polymorphism in the human mu opioid receptor gene alters beta-endorphin binding and activity: possible implications for opiate addiction. *Proc Natl Acad Sci U S A*. 1998 Aug 4;95(16):9608–9613. doi: 10.1073/pnas.95.16.9608. PMID: 9689128; PMCID: PMC21386.

168. Ren ZY, Xu XQ, Bao YP, He J, Shi L, Deng JH, Gao XJ, Tang HL, Wang YM, Lu L. The impact of genetic variation on sensitivity to opioid analgesics in patients with postoperative pain: a systematic review and meta-analysis. *Pain Physician*. 2015 Mar–Apr;18(2):131–152. PMID: 25794200.

169. Li ZX, Ye F, Li WY, Bao YP, Cheng YC, Song ZW, Zhao RS, Ren ZY. The effect of genetic variation on the sensitivity to opioid analgesics in patients with postoperative pain: an updated meta-analysis. *Pain Physician*. 2023 Sep;26(5):E467–E485. PMID: 37774182.

170. Manini AF, Jacobs MM, Vlahov D, Hurd YL. Opioid receptor polymorphism a118g associated with clinical severity in a drug overdose population. *J Med Toxicol*. 2013 Jun;9(2):148–154. doi: 10.1007/s13181-012-0286-3. PMID: 23318993; PMCID: PMC3648633.

171. https://www.fda.gov/drugs/science-and-research-drugs/table-pharmacogenomic-biomarkers-drug-labeling. Accessed October 30, 2023.

172. Fuentes AV, Pineda MD, Venkata KCN. Comprehension of top 200 prescribed drugs in the US as a resource for pharmacy teaching, training and practice. *Pharmacy* (Basel). 2018 May 14;6(2):43. doi: 10.3390/pharmacy6020043. PMID: 29757930; PMCID: PMC6025009.

173. While the commonly used term of "poor metabolizer" in this area of labeling/literature certainly expresses the relatively low capacity for metabolism of a drug, we would point out that the terminology seems to unfairly frame the level of function of detoxification organs based on their capacity to biotransform chemicals not generally innate to their natural environment.

174. https://www.fda.gov/industry/prescription-drug-user-fee-amendments/pdufa-legislation-and-background. Accessed October 19, 2022.

175. Guideline for industry: dose-response information to support drug registration. International Conference on Harmonisation of Technical Requirements for the Registration of Pharmaceuticals for Human Use. 1994. https://www.fda.gov/media/71279/download. Accessed October 19, 2022.

176. Frank C, Himmelstein DU, Woolhandler S, Bor DH, Wolfe SM, Heymann O, Zallman L, Lasser KE. Era of faster FDA drug approval has also seen increased black-box warnings and market withdrawals. *Health Aff* (Millwood). 2014;33(8):1453–1459.

177. Steering Committee of the Physicians' Health Study Research Group. Final report on the aspirin component of the ongoing Physicians' Health Study. *N Engl J Med*. 1989 Jul 20;321(3):129–135. doi: 10.1056/NEJM198907203210301. PMID: 2664509.

178. https://www.accessdata.fda.gov/scripts/cdrh/cfdocs/cfcfr/cfrsearch.cfm?fr=343.80#:~:text=Vascular%20Indications%20(Ischemic%20Stroke%2C%20TIA,the%20brain%20due%20to%20fibrin. Accessed October 10, 2023.

179. US Preventive Services Task Force; Davidson KW, Barry MJ, Mangione CM, Cabana M, Chelmow D, Coker TR, Davis EM, Donahue KE, Jaén CR, Krist AH, Kubik M, Li L, Ogedegbe G, Pbert L, Ruiz JM, Stevermer J, Tseng CW, Wong JB. Aspirin use to prevent cardiovascular disease: US preventive services task force recommendation statement. *JAMA*. 2022 Apr 26;327(16):1577–1584. doi: 10.1001/jama.2022.4983. PMID: 35471505.

180. Campbell CL, Smyth S, Montalescot G, Steinhubl SR. Aspirin dose for the prevention of cardiovascular disease: a systematic review. *JAMA*. 2007 May 9;297(18):2018–2024. doi: 10.1001/jama.297.18.2018. PMID: 17488967.

181. Campbell CL, Smyth S, Montalescot G, Steinhubl SR. Aspirin dose for the prevention of cardiovascular disease: a systematic review. *JAMA*. 2007 May 9;297(18):2018–2024. doi: 10.1001/jama.297.18.2018. PMID: 17488967.

182. Campbell CL, Smyth S, Montalescot G, Steinhubl SR. Aspirin dose for the prevention of cardiovascular disease: a systematic review. *JAMA*. 2007 May 9;297(18):2018–2024. doi: 10.1001/jama.297.18.2018. PMID: 17488967.

183. Skydel JJ, Zhang AD, Dhruva SS, Ross JS, Wallach JD. US Food and Drug Administration utilization of postmarketing requirements and postmarketing commitments, 2009–2018. *Clin Trials*. 2021;18(4):488–499. doi:10.1177/17407745211005044.

184. Resnik DB. Beyond post-marketing research and MedWatch: long-term studies of drug risks. *Drug Des Devel Ther*. 2007;1:1–5. doi:10.2147/dddt.s2352.

185. DAD Study Group, Friis-Møller N, Reiss P, Sabin CA, Weber R, Monforte Ad, El-Sadr W, Thiébaut R, De Wit S, Kirk O, Fontas E, Law MG, Phillips A, Lundgren JD. Class of antiretroviral drugs and the risk of myocardial infarction. *N Engl J Med*. 2007 Apr 26;356(17):1723–1735. doi: 10.1056/NEJMoa062744. PMID: 17460226.

186. Breitinger, HG. Drug synergy-mechanisms and methods of analysis, toxicity and drug testing. In: Acree W, ed. *Toxicity and Drug Testing*. InTech;2012. 143–166. https://www.academia.edu/25545117/Drug_Synergy_Mechanisms_and_Methods_of_Analysis. Accessed October 12, 2022.

187. Zhou X, Seto SW, Chang D, Kiat H, Razmovski-Naumovski V, Chan K, Bensoussan A. Synergistic effects of Chinese herbal medicine: a comprehensive review of methodology and current research. *Front Pharmacol*. 2016;7:201.

188. Wang D, Calabrese EJ, Lian B, Lin Z, Calabrese V. Hormesis as a mechanistic approach to understanding herbal treatments in traditional Chinese medicine. *Pharmacol Ther*. 2018;184:42–50.

189. Liang X, Chen X, Liang Q, Zhang H, Hu P, Wang Y, Luo G. Metabonomic study of Chinese medicine Shuanglong formula as an effective treatment for myocardial infarction in rats. *J Proteome Res*. 2011;10(2):790-9.

190. Xu R, Wu J, Zhang X, Zou X, Li C, Wang H, Yuan M, Chen M, Sun Q, Liu S. Modified Bu-Zhong-Yi-Qi decoction synergies with 5 fluorouracile inhibits gastric cancer progress via PD-1/PD- L1-dependent T cell immunization. *Pharmacol Res*. 2020;152:104623.

191. Bhutani MK, Bishnoi M, Kulkarni SK. Anti-depressant like effect of curcumin and its combination with piperine in unpredictable chronic stress-induced behavioral, biochemical and neurochemical changes. *Pharmacol Biochem Behav*. 2009;92(1):39–43.

192. Panahi Y, Badeli R, Karami GR, Sahebkar A. Investigation of the efficacy of adjunctive therapy with bioavailability-boosted curcuminoids in major depressive disorder. *Phytother Res*. 2015;29(1):17–21.

193. Prakash UN, Srinivasan K. Beneficial influence of dietary spices on the ultrastructure and fluidity of the intestinal brush border in rats. *Br J Nutr*. 2010;104(1):31–39.

194. Khajuria A, Thusu N, Zutshi U. Piperine modulates permeability characteristics of intestine by inducing alterations in membrane dynamics: influence on brush border membrane fluidity, ultrastructure and enzyme kinetics. *Phytomedicine*. 2002;9(3):224–231.

195. Zhang W, Lim LY. Effects of spice constituents on P-glycoprotein-mediated transport and CYP3A4-mediated metabolism in vitro. *Drug Metab Dispos*. 2008;36(7):1283–1290.

196. Prakash UN, Srinivasan K. Enhanced intestinal uptake of iron, zinc and calcium in rats fed pungent spice principles—piperine, capsaicin and ginger (*Zingiber officinale*). *J Trace Elem Med Biol*. 2013;27(3):184–190.

197. Maharao N, Venitz J, Gerk PM. Use of generally recognized as safe or dietary compounds to inhibit buprenorphine metabolism: potential to improve buprenorphine oral bioavailability. *Biopharm Drug Dispos*. 2019;40(1):18–31.

198. Lambert JD, Hong J, Kim DH, Mishin VM, Yang CS. Piperine enhances the bioavailability of the tea polyphenol (-)-epigallocatechin-3-gallate in mice. *J Nutr*. 2004;134(8):1948–1952.

199. Tsuchiya Y, Fujita R, Saitou A, Wajima N, Aizawa F, Iinuma A. [6]-gingerol induces electrogenic sodium absorption in the rat colon via the capsaicin receptor TRPV1. *J Nutr Sci Vitaminol* (Tokyo). 2014;60(6):403–407.

200. Watanabe T, Terada Y. Food compounds activating thermosensitive TRP channels in Asian herbal and medicinal foods. *J Nutr Sci Vitaminol* (Tokyo). 2015;61 Suppl:S86–88.

201. Nakhaee S, Dastjerdi M, Roumi H, Mehrpour O, Farrokhfall K. N-acetylcysteine dose-dependently improves the analgesic effect of acetaminophen on the rat hot plate test. *BMC Pharmacol Toxicol.* 2021;22(1):4.

202. Violi, Francesco MD; Lip, Gregory YH MD; Pignatelli, Pasquale MD; Pastori, Daniele MD. Interaction between dietary vitamin K intake and anticoagulation by vitamin K antagonists: Is it really true? *Medicine.* 2016;95(10):p e2895.

203. Volak LP, Hanley MJ, Masse G, Hazarika S, Harmatz JS, Badmaev V, Majeed M, Greenblatt DJ, Court MH. Effect of an herbal extract containing curcumin and piperine on midazolam, flurbiprofen and paracetamol (acetaminophen) pharmacokinetics in healthy volunteers. *Br J Clin Pharmacol.* 2013 Feb;75(2):450–462. doi: 10.1111/j.1365-2125.2012.04364.x. PMID: 22725836; PMCID: PMC3579260.

204. Volak LP, Ghirmai S, Cashman JR, Court MH. Curcuminoids inhibit multiple human cytochromes P450, UDP-glucuronosyltransferase, and sulfotransferase enzymes, whereas piperine is a relatively selective CYP3A4 inhibitor. *Drug Metab Dispos.* 2008 Aug;36(8):1594–1605. doi: 10.1124/dmd.108.020552. Epub 2008 May 14. PMID: 18480186; PMCID: PMC2574793.

205. Ha H, Lee JK, Lee HY, Seo C-S, Kim J-H, Lee M-Y, Koh W-S, Shin HK. Evaluation of safety of the herbal formula Ojeok-san: acute and sub-chronic toxicity studies in rats. *Journal of Ethnopharmacology.* 2010;131(2):410–416.

206. Ko Y, Go HY, Han IS, et al. Efficacy and safety of Ojeok-san in Korean female patients with cold hypersensitivity in the hands and feet: study protocol for a randomized, double-blinded, placebo-controlled, multicenter pilot study. *Trials.* 2018:19(62).

207. Park SI, Park JY, Park MJ, Yim SV, Kim BH. Effects of Ojeok-san on the pharmacokinetics of celecoxib at steady-state in healthy volunteers. *Basic Clin Pharmacol Toxicol*. 2018 Jul;123(1):51–57. doi: 10.1111/bcpt.12971. Epub 2018 Mar 15. PMID: 29377603.

208. Toh DS, Limenta LM, Yee JY, Wang LZ, Goh BC, Murray M, Lee EJ. Effect of mushroom diet on pharmacokinetics of gabapentin in healthy Chinese subjects. *Br J Clin Pharmacol*. 2014 Jul;78(1):129–134. doi: 10.1111/bcp.12273. PMID: 24168107; PMCID: PMC4168387.

209. Gurley BJ, Swain A, Hubbard MA, Hartsfield F, Thaden J, Williams DK, Gentry WB, Tong Y. Supplementation with goldenseal (*Hydrastis canadensis*), but not kava kava (*Piper methysticum*), inhibits human CYP3A activity in vivo. *Clin Pharmacol Ther*. 2008 Jan;83(1):61–69. doi: 10.1038/sj.clpt.6100222. Epub 2007 May 9. PMID: 17495878.

210. Gurley BJ, Gardner SF, Hubbard MA, Williams DK, Gentry WB, Khan IA, Shah A. In vivo effects of goldenseal, kava kava, black cohosh, and valerian on human cytochrome P450 1A2, 2D6, 2E1, and 3A4/5 phenotypes. *Clin Pharmacol Ther*. 2005 May;77(5):415–426. doi: 10.1016/j.clpt.2005.01.009. PMID: 15900287; PMCID: PMC1894911.

211. Nguyen JT, Tian DD, Tanna RS, Hadi DL, Bansal S, Calamia JC, Arian CM, Shireman LM, Molnár B, Horváth M, Kellogg JJ, Layton ME, White JR, Cech NB, Boyce RD, Unadkat JD, Thummel KE, Paine MF. Assessing transporter-mediated natural product-drug interactions via in vitro-in vivo extrapolation: clinical evaluation with a probe cocktail. *Clin Pharmacol Ther*. 2021 May;109(5):1342–1352. doi: 10.1002/cpt.2107. Epub 2020 Dec 23. PMID: 33174626; PMCID: PMC8058163.

212. Gurley BJ, Swain A, Barone GW, Williams DK, Breen P, Yates CR, Stuart LB, Hubbard MA, Tong Y, Cheboyina S. Effect of goldenseal (*Hydrastis canadensis*) and kava kava (*Piper methysticum*) supplementation on digoxin pharmacokinetics in humans. *Drug Metab Dispos*. 2007 Feb;35(2):240–245. doi: 10.1124/dmd.106.012708. Epub 2006 Nov 1. PMID: 17079360; PMCID: PMC1868501.

213. Zhou S, Chan E, Pan SQ, Huang M, Lee EJ. Pharmacokinetic interactions of drugs with St John's wort. *J Psychopharmacol*. 2004 Jun;18(2):262–276. doi: 10.1177/0269881104042632. PMID: 15260917.

214. Johne A, Schmider J, Brockmöller J, Stadelmann AM, Störmer E, Bauer S, Scholler G, Langheinrich M, Roots I. Decreased plasma levels of amitriptyline and its metabolites on comedication with an extract from St. John's wort (*Hypericum perforatum*). *J Clin Psychopharmacol*. 2002 Feb;22(1):46–54. doi: 10.1097/00004714-200202000-00008. PMID: 11799342.

215. Rey JM, Walter G. Hypericum perforatum (St John's wort) in depression: pest or blessing? *Med J Aust*. 1998 Dec 7–21;169(11-12):583–586. doi: 10.5694/j.1326-5377.1998.tb123424.x. PMID: 9887899.

216. Johne A, Brockmöller J, Bauer S, Maurer A, Langheinrich M, Roots I. Pharmacokinetic interaction of digoxin with an herbal extract from St John's wort (*Hypericum perforatum*). *Clin Pharmacol Ther*. 1999 Oct;66(4):338–345. doi: 10.1053/cp.1999.v66.a101944. PMID: 10546917.

217. Wang Z, Hamman MA, Huang SM, Lesko LJ, Hall SD. Effect of St John's wort on the pharmacokinetics of fexofenadine. *Clin Pharmacol Ther*. 2002 Jun;71(6):414–420. doi: 10.1067/mcp.2002.124080. PMID: 12087344.

218. Xu H, Williams KM, Liauw WS, Murray M, Day RO, McLachlan AJ. Effects of St John's wort and CYP2C9 genotype on the pharmacokinetics and pharmacodynamics of gliclazide. *Br J Pharmacol*. 2008 Apr;153(7):1579–1586. doi: 10.1038/sj.bjp.0707685. Epub 2008 Jan 21. PMID: 18204476; PMCID: PMC2437900.

219. Piscitelli SC, Burstein AH, Chaitt D, Alfaro RM, Falloon J. Indinavir concentrations and St John's wort. *Lancet*. 2000 Feb 12;355(9203):547–548. doi: 10.1016/S0140-6736(99)05712-8. Erratum in: Lancet. 2001 Apr 14;357(9263):1210. PMID: 10683007.

220. Eich-Höchli D, Oppliger R, Golay KP, Baumann P, Eap CB. Methadone maintenance treatment and St. John's Wort—a case report. *Pharmacopsychiatry*. 2003 Jan;36(1):35–37. doi: 10.1055/s-2003-38090. PMID: 12649774.

221. Wang Z, Gorski JC, Hamman MA, Huang SM, Lesko LJ, Hall SD. The effects of St John's wort (*Hypericum perforatum*) on human cytochrome P450 activity. *Clin Pharmacol Ther*. 2001 Oct;70(4):317–326. PMID: 11673747.

222. de Maat MM, Hoetelmans RM, Math t RA, van Gorp EC, Meenhorst PL, Mulder JW, Beijnen JH. Drug interaction between St John's wort and nevirapine. *AIDS*. 2001 Feb 16;15(3):420–421. doi: 10.1097/00002030-200102160-00019. PMID: 11273226.

223. Nieminen TH, Hagelberg NM, Saari TI, Neuvonen M, Laine K, Neuvonen PJ, Olkkola KT. St John's wort greatly reduces the concentrations of oral oxycodone. *Eur J Pain.* 2010 Sep;14(8):854–859. doi: 10.1016/j.ejpain.2009.12.007. Epub 2010 Jan 27. PMID: 20106684.

224. Maurer A, Johne A, Bauer S, Brockmoller F, Conath I, Roots M, Langheinrich M, Hubner WD. Interaction of St. John's wort extract with phenprocoumon [Abstract]. *European Journal of Clinical Pharmacology.* 1999;55:A22.

225. Sugimoto K, Ohmori M, Tsuruoka S, Nishiki K, Kawaguchi A, Harada K, Arakawa M, Sakamoto K, Masada M, Miyamori I, Fujimura A. Different effects of St John's wort on the pharmacokinetics of simvastatin and pravastatin. *Clin Pharmacol Ther.* 2001 Dec;70(6):518–524. doi: 10.1067/mcp.2001.120025. PMID: 11753267.

226. Mai I, Störmer E, Bauer S, Krüger H, Budde K, Roots I. Impact of St John's wort treatment on the pharmacokinetics of tacrolimus and mycophenolic acid in renal transplant patients. *Nephrol Dial Transplant.* 2003 Apr;18(4):819–822. doi: 10.1093/ndt/gfg002. PMID: 12637655.

227. Nebel A, Schneider BJ, Baker RK, Kroll DJ. Potential metabolic interaction between St. John's wort and theophylline. *Ann Pharmacother.* 1999 Apr;33(4):502. doi: 10.1345/aph.18252. PMID: 10332544.

228. Yue QY, Bergquist C, Gerdén B. Safety of St John's wort (*Hypericum perforatum*). *Lancet.* 2000 Feb 12;355(9203):576–577. doi: 10.1016/S0140-6736(05)73227-X. PMID: 10683030.

229. Jiang X, Williams KM, Liauw WS, Ammit AJ, Roufogalis BD, Duke CC, Day RO, McLachlan AJ. Effect of St John's wort and ginseng on the pharmacokinetics and pharmacodynamics of warfarin in healthy subjects. *Br J Clin Pharmacol*. 2004 May;57(5):592–599. doi: 10.1111/j.1365-2125.2003.02051.x. Erratum in: *Br J Clin Pharmacol*. 2004 Jul;58(1):102. PMID: 15089812; PMCID: PMC1884493.

230. Jiang X, Blair EY, McLachlan AJ. Investigation of the effects of herbal medicines on warfarin response in healthy subjects: a population pharmacokinetic-pharmacodynamic modeling approach. *J Clin Pharmacol*. 2006 Nov;46(11):1370–1378. doi: 10.1177/0091270006292124. PMID: 17050802.

231. Loughren MJ, Kharasch ED, Kelton-Rehkopf MC, Syrjala KL, Shen DD. Influence of St. John's wort on intravenous fentanyl pharmacokinetics, pharmacodynamics, and clinical effects: a randomized clinical trial. *Anesthesiology*. 2020 Mar;132(3):491–503. doi: 10.1097/ALN.0000000000003065. PMID: 31794512; PMCID: PMC7029805.

232. Zhou S, Yung Chan S, Cher Goh B, Chan E, Duan W, Huang M, McLeod HL. Mechanism-based inhibition of cytochrome P450 3A4 by therapeutic drugs. *Clin Pharmacokinet*. 2005;44(3):279–304. doi: 10.2165/00003088-200544030-00005. PMID: 15762770.

233. Lynch T, Price A. The effect of cytochrome P450 metabolism on drug response, interactions, and adverse effects. Am Fam Physician. 2007 Aug 1;76(3):391–396. PMID: 17708140.

234. Wang D, Zhao T, Zhao S, Chen J, Dou T, Ge G, Wang C, Sun H, Liu K, Meng Q, Wu J. Substrate-dependent inhibition of hypericin on human carboxylesterase 2: implications for herb-drug combination. *Curr Drug Metab*. 2022;23(1):38–44. doi: 10.2174/13892002236662 20202093303. PMID: 35114918.

235. Kim TE, Ha N, Kim Y, Kim H, Lee JW, Jeon JY, Kim MG. Effect of epigallocatechin-3-gallate, major ingredient of green tea, on the pharmacokinetics of rosuvastatin in healthy volunteers. *Drug Des Devel Ther.* 2017 May 9;11:1409–1416. doi: 10.2147/DDDT.S130050. PMID: 28533679; PMCID: PMC5431696.

236. Abdelkawy KS, Abdelaziz RM, Abdelmageed AM, Donia AM, El-Khodary NM. Effects of green tea extract on atorvastatin pharmacokinetics in healthy volunteers. *Eur J Drug Metab Pharmacokinet.* 2020 Jun;45(3):351–360. doi: 10.1007/s13318-020-00608-6. PMID: 31997084.

237. Misaka S, Abe O, Ono T, Ono Y, Ogata H, Miura I, Shikama Y, Fromm MF, Yabe H, Shimomura K. Effects of single green tea ingestion on pharmacokinetics of nadolol in healthy volunteers. *Br J Clin Pharmacol.* 2020 Nov;86(11):2314–2318. doi: 10.1111/bcp.14315. Epub 2020 May 12. PMID: 32320490; PMCID: PMC7576630.

238. Misaka S, Ono Y, Uchida A, Ono T, Abe O, Ogata H, Sato H, Suzuki M, Onoue S, Shikama Y, Shimomura K. Impact of green tea catechin ingestion on the pharmacokinetics of lisinopril in healthy volunteers. *Clin Transl Sci.* 2021 Mar;14(2):476–480. doi: 10.1111/cts.12905. Epub 2020 Oct 22. PMID: 33048477; PMCID: PMC7993260.

239. Veerman GDM, van der Werff SC, Koolen SLW, Miedema JR, Oomen-de Hoop E, van der Mark SC, Chandoesing PP, de Bruijn P, Wijsenbeek MS, Mathijssen RHJ. The influence of green tea extract on nintedanib's bioavailability in patients with pulmonary fibrosis. *Biomed Pharmacother.* 2022 Jul;151:113101. doi: 10.1016/j.biopha.2022.113101. Epub 2022 May 17. PMID: 35594703.

240. Malati CY, Robertson SM, Hunt JD, Chairez C, Alfaro RM, Kovacs JA, Penzak SR. Influence of Panax ginseng on cytochrome P450 (CYP)3A and P-glycoprotein (P-gp) activity in healthy participants. *J Clin Pharmacol*. 2012 Jun;52(6):932–939. doi: 10.1177/0091270011407194. Epub 2011 Jun 6. PMID: 21646440; PMCID: PMC3523324.

241. Calderón MM, Chairez CL, Gordon LA, Alfaro RM, Kovacs JA, Penzak SR. Influence of Panax ginseng on the steady state pharmacokinetic profile of lopinavir-ritonavir in healthy volunteers. *Pharmacotherapy*. 2014 Nov;34(11):1151–1158. doi: 10.1002/phar.1473. Epub 2014 Aug 20. PMID: 25142999; PMCID: PMC5466349.

242. https://www.accessdata.fda.gov/drugsatfda_docs/label/2007/021226s018lbl.pdf. Accessed February 21, 2023.

243. Lee SH, Ahn YM, Ahn SY, Doo HK, Lee BC. Interaction between warfarin and Panax ginseng in ischemic stroke patients. *J Altern Complement Med*. 2008 Jul;14(6):715–721. doi: 10.1089/acm.2007.0799. PMID: 18637764.

244. Jiang X, Blair EY, McLachlan AJ. Investigation of the effects of herbal medicines on warfarin response in healthy subjects: a population pharmacokinetic-pharmacodynamic modeling approach. *J Clin Pharmacol*. 2006 Nov;46(11):1370–1378. doi: 10.1177/0091270006292124. PMID: 17050802.

245. Wang W, Yang L, Song L, Guo M, Li C, Yang B, Wang M, Kou N, Gao J, Qu H, Ma Y, Xue M, Shi D. Combination of *Panax notoginseng* saponins and aspirin potentiates platelet inhibition with alleviated gastric injury via modulating arachidonic acid metabolism. *Biomed Pharmacother*. 2021 Feb;134:111165. doi: 10.1016/j.biopha.2020.111165. Epub 2020 Dec 25. PMID: 33370633.

246. Yuan CS, Wei G, Dey L, Karrison T, Nahlik L, Maleckar S, Kasza K, Ang-Lee M, Moss J. Brief communication: American ginseng reduces warfarin's effect in healthy patients: a randomized, controlled trial. *Ann Intern Med*. 2004 Jul 6;141(1):23–27. doi: 10.7326/0003-4819-141-1-200407060-00011. PMID: 15238367.

247. Robertson SM, Davey RT, Voell J, Formentini E, Alfaro RM, Penzak SR. Effect of *Ginkgo biloba* extract on lopinavir, midazolam and fexofenadine pharmacokinetics in healthy subjects. *Curr Med Res Opin*. 2008 Feb;24(2):591-9. doi: 10.1185/030079908x260871. PMID: 18205997.

248. Uchida S, Yamada H, Li XD, Maruyama S, Ohmori Y, Oki T, Watanabe H, Umegaki K, Ohashi K, Yamada S. Effects of *Ginkgo biloba* extract on pharmacokinetics and pharmacodynamics of tolbutamide and midazolam in healthy volunteers. *J Clin Pharmacol*. 2006 Nov;46(11):1290–1298. doi: 10.1177/0091270006292628. PMID: 17050793.

249. Yoshioka M, Ohnishi N, Koishi T, Obata Y, Nakagawa M, Matsumoto T, Tagagi K, Takara K, Ohkuni T, Yokoyama T, Kuroda K. Studies on interactions between functional foods or dietary supplements and medicines. IV. Effects of ginkgo biloba leaf extract on the pharmacokinetics and pharmacodynamics of nifedipine in healthy volunteers. *Biol Pharm Bull*. 2004 Dec;27(12):2006ü2009. doi: 10.1248/bpb.27.2006. PMID: 15577221.

250. Yin OQ, Tomlinson B, Waye MM, Chow AH, Chow MS. Pharmacogenetics and herb-drug interactions: experience with Ginkgo biloba and omeprazole. *Pharmacogenetics*. 2004 Dec;14(12):841–850. doi: 10.1097/00008571-200412000-00007. PMID: 15608563.

251. Gorski JC, Huang SM, Pinto A, Hamman MA, Hilligoss JK, Zaheer NA, Desai M, Miller M, Hall SD. The effect of echinacea (*Echinacea purpurea* root) on cytochrome P450 activity in vivo. *Clin Pharmacol Ther*. 2004 Jan;75(1):89–100. doi: 10.1016/j.clpt.2003.09.013. PMID: 14749695.

252. Moltó J, Valle M, Miranda C, Cedeño S, Negredo E, Barbanoj MJ, Clotet B. Herb-drug interaction between *Echinacea purpurea* and darunavir-ritonavir in HIV-infected patients. *Antimicrob Agents Chemother*. 2011 Jan;55(1):326–330. doi: 10.1128/AAC.01082-10. Epub 2010 Nov 15. PMID: 21078942; PMCID: PMC3019656.

253. Abdul MI, Jiang X, Williams KM, Day RO, Roufogalis BD, Liauw WS, Xu H, Matthias A, Lehmann RP, McLachlan AJ. Pharmacokinetic and pharmacodynamic interactions of echinacea and policosanol with warfarin in healthy subjects. *Br J Clin Pharmacol*. 2010 May;69(5):508–515. doi: 10.1111/j.1365-2125.2010.03620.x. PMID: 20573086; PMCID: PMC2856051.

254. Ellis GR, Stephens MR. Untitled (photograph and a brief case report). *BMJ*. 1999;319(7210):650.

255. Page RL 2nd, Lawrence JD. Potentiation of warfarin by dong quai. *Pharmacotherapy*. 1999 Jul;19(7):870–876. doi: 10.1592/phco.19.10.870.31558. PMID: 10417036.

256. Houben RJ, Brunt K. Determination of glycoalkaloids in potato tubers by reversed-phase high performance liquid chromatography. *Journal of Chromatography A*. 1994; 661(1-2):169–174.

257. Roddick JG, Melchers G. Steroidal glycoalkaloid content of potato, tomato and their somatic hybrids. *Theor Appl Genet*. 1985 Sep;70(6):655–660. doi: 10.1007/BF00252292. PMID: 24253124.

258. Dzakovich MP, Hartman JL, Cooperstone JL. A high-throughput extraction and analysis method for steroidal glycoalkaloids in tomato. *Front Plant Sci*. 2020 Jun 18;11:767. doi:10.3389/fpls.2020.00767.

259. Mennella G, Lo Scalzo R, Fibiani M, D'Alessandro A, Francese G, Toppino L, Acciarri N, de Almeida AE, Rotino GL. Chemical and bioactive quality traits during fruit ripening in eggplant (*S. melongena* L.) and allied species. *J Agric Food Chem*. 2012 Nov 28;60(47):11821–11831. doi: 10.1021/jf3037424. Epub 2012 Nov 19. PMID: 23134376.

260. Jones PG, Fenwick GR. The glycoalkaloid content of some edible solanaceous fruits and potato products. *J Sci Food Agric*. 1981 Apr;32(4):419–421. doi: 10.1002/jsfa.2740320418. PMID: 7242021.

261. Peeples A, Dalvi RR. Toxic alkaloids and their interaction with microsomal cytochrome P-450 in vitro. *J Appl Toxicol*. 1982 Dec;2(6):300–302. doi: 10.1002/jat.2550020607. PMID: 7185909.

262. Bushway RJ, Savage SA, Ferguson BS. Inhibition of acetyl cholinesterase by solanaceous glycoalkaloids and alkaloids. *American Potato Journal*. 1987;64:409–413. https://doi.org/10.1007/BF02853703.

263. Lelario F, De Maria S, Rivelli AR, Russo D, Milella L, Bufo SA, Scrano L. A complete survey of glycoalkaloids using LC-FTI-CR-MS and IRMPD in a commercial variety and a local landrace of eggplant (*Solanum melongena* L.) and their anticholinesterase and antioxidant activities. *Toxins* (Basel). 2019 Apr 19;11(4):230. doi: 10.3390/toxins11040230. PMID: 31010145; PMCID: PMC6521288.

264. McGehee DS, Krasowski MD, Fung DL, Wilson B, Gronert GA, Moss J. Cholinesterase inhibition by potato glycoalkaloids slows mivacurium metabolism. *Anesthesiology*. 2000 Aug;93(2):510–519. doi: 10.1097/00000542-200008000-00031. PMID: 10910502.

265. Harvey MH, McMillan M, Morgan MR, Chan HW. Solanidine is present in sera of healthy individuals and in amounts dependent on their dietary potato consumption. *Hum Toxicol*. 1985 Mar;4(2):187–194. doi: 10.1177/096032718500400209. PMID: 4007882.

266. Hellenäs KE, Nyman A, Slanina P, Lööf L, Gabrielsson J. Determination of potato glycoalkaloids and their aglycone in blood serum by high-performance liquid chromatography. Application to pharmacokinetic studies in humans. *J Chromatogr*. 1992 Jan 3;573(1):69–78. doi: 10.1016/0378-4347(92)80476-7. PMID: 1564109.

267. Guo Y, Chen Y, Tan ZR, Klaassen CD, Zhou HH. Repeated administration of berberine inhibits cytochromes P450 in humans. *Eur J Clin Pharmacol*. 2012 Feb;68(2):213–217. doi: 10.1007/s00228-011-1108-2. Epub 2011 Aug 26. PMID: 21870106; PMCID: PMC4898966.

268. Sarraf M, Beig Babaei A, Naji-Tabasi S. Investigating functional properties of barberry species: an overview. *J Sci Food Agric*. 2019 Sep;99(12):5255–5269. doi: 10.1002/jsfa.9804. Epub 2019 Jun 27. PMID: 31077383.

269. Katare AK, Singh B, Shukla P, Gupta S, Singh B, Yalamanchili K, Kulshrestha N, Bhanwaria R, Sharma AK, Sharma S, Sneha, Mindala DP, Roy S, Kalgotra R. Rapid determination and optimization of berberine from Himalayan *Berberis lycium* by soxhlet apparatus using CCD-RSM and its quality control as a potential candidate for COVID-19. *Nat Prod Res*. 2022 Feb;36(3):868–873. doi: 10.1080/14786419.2020.1806274. Epub 2020 Aug 13. PMID: 32787584.

270. Roy NS, Choi IY, Um T, Jeon MJ, Kim BY, Kim YD, Yu JK, Kim S, Kim NS. Gene expression and isoform identification of PacBio full-length cDNA sequences for berberine biosynthesis in *Berberis koreana*. *Plants* (Basel). 2021 Jun 28;10(7):1314. doi: 10.3390/plants10071314. PMID: 34203474; PMCID: PMC8308982.

271. Ji X, Li Y, Liu H, Yan Y, Li J. Determination of the alkaloid content in different parts of some Mahonia plants by HPCE. *Pharm Acta Helv*. 2000 Apr;74(4):387–391. doi: 10.1016/s0031-6865(99)00061-8. PMID: 10812938.

272. Galle K, Müller-Jakic B, Proebstle A, Jurcic K, Bladt S, Wagner H. Analytical and pharmacological studies on *Mahonia aquifolium*. *Phytomedicine*. 1994 Jun;1(1):59–62. doi: 10.1016/S0944-7113(11)80024-3. PMID: 23195817.

273. Weber HA, Zart MK, Hodges AE, White KD, Barnes SM, Moody LA, Clark AP, Harris RK, Overstreet JD, Smith CS. Method validation for determination of alkaloid content in goldenseal root powder. *J AOAC Int.* 2003 May–Jun;86(3):476–483. PMID: 12852562.

274. He F, Huang YF, Dai W, Qu XY, Lu JG, Lao CC, Luo WH, Sun DM, Wei M, Xiao SY, Xie Y, Liu L, Zhou H. The localization of the alkaloids in *Coptis chinensis* rhizome by time-of-flight secondary ion mass spectrometry. *Front Plant Sci.* 2022 Dec 23;13:1092643. doi: 10.3389/fpls.2022.1092643. PMID: 36618650; PMCID: PMC9816869.

275. Pandey G, Khatoon S, Pandey MM, Rawat AKS. Altitudinal variation of berberine, total phenolics and flavonoid content in *Thalictrum foliolosum* and their correlation with antimicrobial and antioxidant activities. *J Ayurveda Integr Med.* 2018 Jul–Sep;9(3):169–176. doi: 10.1016/j.jaim.2017.02.010. PMID: 29102462; PMCID: PMC6148047.

276. Rojsanga P, Gritsanapan W, Suntornsuk L. Determination of berberine content in the stem extracts of *Coscinium fenestratum* by TLC densitometry. *Med Princ Pract.* 2006;15(5):373–378. doi: 10.1159/000094272. PMID: 16888396.

277. Kim TE, Ha N, Kim Y, Kim H, Lee JW, Jeon JY, Kim MG. Effect of epigallocatechin-3-gallate, major ingredient of green tea, on the pharmacokinetics of rosuvastatin in healthy volunteers. *Drug Des Devel Ther.* 2017 May 9;11:1409–1416. doi: 10.2147/DDDT.S130050. PMID: 28533679; PMCID: PMC5431696.

278. Abdelkawy KS, Abdelaziz RM, Abdelmageed AM, Donia AM, El-Khodary NM. Effects of green tea extract on atorvastatin pharmacokinetics in healthy volunteers. *Eur J Drug Metab Pharmacokinet*. 2020 Jun;45(3):351–360. doi: 10.1007/s13318-020-00608-6. PMID: 31997084.

279. Misaka S, Ono Y, Uchida A, Ono T, Abe O, Ogata H, Sato H, Suzuki M, Onoue S, Shikama Y, Shimomura K. Impact of green tea catechin ingestion on the pharmacokinetics of lisinopril in healthy volunteers. *Clin Transl Sci*. 2021 Mar;14(2):476–480. doi: 10.1111/cts.12905. Epub 2020 Oct 22. PMID: 33048477; PMCID: PMC7993260.

280. Misaka S, Abe O, Ono T, Ono Y, Ogata H, Miura I, Shikama Y, Fromm MF, Yabe H, Shimomura K. Effects of single green tea ingestion on pharmacokinetics of nadolol in healthy volunteers. *Br J Clin Pharmacol*. 2020 Nov;86(11):2314–2318. doi: 10.1111/bcp.14315. Epub 2020 May 12. PMID: 32320490; PMCID: PMC7576630.

281. Veerman GDM, van der Werff SC, Koolen SLW, Miedema JR, Oomen-de Hoop E, van der Mark SC, Chandoesing PP, de Bruijn P, Wijsenbeek MS, Mathijssen RHJ. The influence of green tea extract on nintedanib's bioavailability in patients with pulmonary fibrosis. *Biomed Pharmacother*. 2022 Jul;151:113101. doi: 10.1016/j.biopha.2022.113101. Epub 2022 May 17. PMID: 35594703.

282. Fuhr U, Kummert AL. The fate of naringin in humans: a key to grapefruit juice-drug interactions? *Clin Pharmacol Ther*. 1995 Oct;58(4):365–373. doi: 10.1016/0009-9236(95)90048-9. PMID: 7586927.

283. https://www.fda.gov/drugs/drug-interactions-labeling/drug-development-and-drug-interactions-table-substrates-inhibitors-and-inducers. Accessed March 16, 2023.

284. Bailey DG, Dresser GK, Kreeft JH, Munoz C, Freeman DJ, Bend JR. Grapefruit-felodipine interaction: effect of unprocessed fruit and probable active ingredients. *Clin Pharmacol Ther*. 2000 Nov;68(5):468–477. doi: 10.1067/mcp.2000.110774. PMID: 11103749.

285. Paine MF, Widmer WW, Hart HL, Pusek SN, Beavers KL, Criss AB, Brown SS, Thomas BF, Watkins PB. A furanocoumarin-free grapefruit juice establishes furanocoumarins as the mediators of the grapefruit juice-felodipine interaction. *Am J Clin Nutr*. 2006 May;83(5):1097–1105. doi: 10.1093/ajcn/83.5.1097. Erratum in: *Am J Clin Nutr*. 2006 Jul;84(1):264. PMID: 16685052.

286. Bailey DG, Arnold JM, Munoz C, Spence JD. Grapefruit juice--felodipine interaction: mechanism, predictability, and effect of naringin. *Clin Pharmacol Ther*. 1993 Jun;53(6):637–642. doi: 10.1038/clpt.1993.84. PMID: 8513655.

287. Cvetkovic M, Leake B, Fromm MF, Wilkinson GR, Kim RB. OATP and P-glycoprotein transporters mediate the cellular uptake and excretion of fexofenadine. *Drug Metab Dispos*. 1999 Aug;27(8):866–871. PMID: 10421612.

288. Franke RM, Scherkenbach LA, Sparreboom A. Pharmacogenetics of the organic anion transporting polypeptide 1A2. *Pharmacogenomics*. 2009;10(3):339–344. doi:10.2217/14622416.10.3.339.

289. Dresser GK, Bailey DG, Leake BF, Schwarz UI, Dawson PA, Freeman DJ, Kim RB. Fruit juices inhibit organic anion transporting polypeptide-mediated drug uptake to decrease the oral availability of fexofenadine. *Clin Pharmacol Ther*. 2002 Jan;71(1):11–20. doi: 10.1067/mcp.2002.121152. PMID: 11823753.

290. Bailey DG, Dresser GK, Leake BF, Kim RB. Naringin is a major and selective clinical inhibitor of organic anion-transporting polypeptide 1A2 (OATP1A2) in grapefruit juice. *Clin Pharmacol Ther*. 2007 Apr;81(4):495–502. doi: 10.1038/sj.clpt.6100104. Epub 2007 Feb 14. PMID: 17301733.

291. Grenier J, Fradette C, Morelli G, Merritt GJ, Vranderick M, Ducharme MP. Pomelo juice, but not cranberry juice, affects the pharmacokinetics of cyclosporine in humans. *Clin Pharmacol Ther*. 2006 Mar;79(3):255–262. doi: 10.1016/j.clpt.2005.11.010. Epub 2006 Feb 7. PMID: 16513449.

292. Dugrand-Judek A, Olry A, Hehn A, Costantino G, Ollitrault P, Froelicher Y, et al. The distribution of coumarins and furanocoumarins in citrus species closely matches citrus phylogeny and reflects the organization of biosynthetic pathways. *PLoS ONE*. 2015;10(11): e0142757.

293. Gardana C, Nalin F, Simonetti P. Evaluation of flavonoids and furanocoumarins from *Citrus bergamia* (bergamot) juice and identification of new compounds. *Molecules*. 2008 Sep 18;13(9):2220-8. doi: 10.3390/molecules13092220. PMID: 18830151; PMCID: PMC6244945.

294. Alehaideb Z, Sheriffdeen M, Law FCP. Inhibition of caffeine metabolism by *Apiaceous* and *Rutaceae* families of plant products in humans: *in vivo* and *in vitro* studies. *Front Pharmacol*. 2021 Apr 29;12:641090. doi: 10.3389/fphar.2021.641090. PMID: 33995046; PMCID: PMC8116649.

295. Maish WA, Hampton EM, Whitsett TL, Shepard JD, Lovallo WR. Influence of grapefruit juice on caffeine pharmacokinetics and pharmacodynamics. *Pharmacotherapy*. 1996 Nov–Dec;16(6):1046–1052. PMID: 8947977.

296. Verkerk R, Schreiner M, Krumbein A, Ciska E, Holst B, Rowland I, De Schrijver R, Hansen M, Gerhäuser C, Mithen R, Dekker M. Glucosinolates in Brassica vegetables: the influence of the food supply chain on intake, bioavailability and human health. *Mol Nutr Food Res*. 2009 Sep;53 Suppl 2:S219. doi: 10.1002/mnfr.200800065. PMID: 19035553.

297. Campas-Baypoli ON, Bueno-Solano C, Martínez-Ibarra DM, Camacho-Gil F, Villa-Lerma AG, Rodríguez-Núñez JR, Lóez-Cervantes J, Sánchez-Machado DI. Contenido de sulforafano (1-isotiocianato-4-(metilsulfinil)-butano) en vegetales crucíferos [Sulforaphane (1-isothiocyanato-4-(methylsulfinyl)-butane) content in cruciferous vegetables]. *Arch Latinoam Nutr*. 2009 Mar;59(1):95–100. Spanish. PMID: 19480351.

298. Bradfield CA, Bjeldanes LF. Modification of carcinogen metabolism by indolylic autolysis products of *Brassica oleraceae*. *Adv Exp Med Biol*. 1991;289:153–163. doi: 10.1007/978-1-4899-2626-5_13. PMID: 1897390.

299. Chevolleau S, Gasc N, Rollin P, Tulliez J. Enzymatic, chemical, and thermal breakdown of ³H-labeled glucobrassicin, the parent indole glucosinolate. *J Agric Food Chem*. 1997;45:4290–4296. See also Grose KR, Bjeldanes LF. Oligomerization of indole-3-carbinol in aqueous acid. *Chem Res Toxicol*. 1992 Mar-Apr;5(2):188–193. doi: 10.1021/tx00026a007. PMID: 1643248.

300. Lubelska K, Milczarek M, Modzelewska K, Krzysztoń-Russjan J, Fronczyk K, Wiktorska K. Interactions between drugs and sulforaphane modulate the drug metabolism enzymatic system. *Pharmacol Rep*. 2012;64(5):1243–1252. doi: 10.1016/s1734-1140(12)70920-9. PMID: 23238480.

301. Shankar E, Goel A, Gupta K, Gupta S. Plant flavone apigenin: An emerging anticancer agent. *Curr Pharmacol Rep*. 2017;3(6):423–446. doi:10.1007/s40495-017-0113-2.

302. Svehlíková V, Wang S, Jakubíková J, Williamson G, Mithen R, Bao Y. Interactions between sulforaphane and apigenin in the induction of UGT1A1 and GSTA1 in CaCo-2 cells. *Carcinogenesis*. 2004 Sep;25(9):1629–1637. doi: 10.1093/carcin/bgh169. Epub 2004 Apr 16. PMID: 15090468.

303. Katchamart S, Stresser DM, Dehal SS, Kupfer D, Williams DE. Concurrent flavin-containing monooxygenase down-regulation and cytochrome P-450 induction by dietary indoles in rat: implications for drug-drug interaction. *Drug Metab Dispos*. 2000 Aug;28(8):930–936. PMID: 10901703.

304. Unger JM, Vaidya R, Hershman DL, Minasian LM, Fleury ME. Systematic review and meta-analysis of the magnitude of structural, clinical, and physician and patient barriers to cancer clinical trial participation. *J Natl Cancer Inst*. 2019 Mar 1;111(3):245–255. doi: 10.1093/jnci/djy221. PMID: 30856272; PMCID: PMC6410951.

305. Carlisle B, Kimmelman J, Ramsay T, MacKinnon N. Unsuccessful trial accrual and human subjects protections: an empirical analysis of recently closed trials. *Clin Trials*. 2015 Feb;12(1):77–83. doi: 10.1177/1740774514558307. Epub 2014 Dec 4. PMID: 25475878; PMCID: PMC4516407.

306. Baldi I, Lanera C, Berchialla P, Gregori D. Early termination of cardiovascular trials as a consequence of poor accrual: analysis of ClinicalTrials.gov 2006-2015. *BMJ Open*. 2017 Jun 15;7(6):e013482. doi: 10.1136/bmjopen-2016-013482. PMID: 28619765; PMCID: PMC5577897.

307. Smalley E. Clinical trials go virtual, big pharma dives in. *Nat Biotechnol*. 2018 Jul 6;36(7):561–562. doi: 10.1038/nbt0718-561. PMID: 29979664. Quotation attributed to Novartis Chief Digital Officer, Bertrand Bodson.

308. Ioannidis JP. Contradicted and initially stronger effects in highly cited clinical research. *JAMA*. 2005 Jul 13;294(2):218–228. doi: 10.1001/jama.294.2.218. PMID: 16014596.

309. 2015–2019. Drug Trials Snapshots. Summary Report. Five-year summary and analysis of clinical trial participation and demographics. U.S. Food and Drug Administration. https://www.fda.gov/media/143592/download?attachment. Accessed January 8, 2024.

310. https://www.census.gov/quickfacts/fact/table/US/POP010220#POP010220. Accessed January 8, 2024.

311. 2015–2019. Drug Trials Snapshots. Summary Report. Five-year summary and analysis of clinical trial participation and demographics. U.S. Food and Drug Administration. https://www.fda.gov/media/143592/download?attachment. Accessed January 8, 2024.

312. Diversity plans to improve enrollment of participants from underrepresented racial and ethnic populations in clinical trials Guidance for Industry. U.S. Department of Health and Human Services. Food and Drug Administration. April 2022. https://www.fda.gov/media/157635/download. Accessed January 17, 2023.

313. 2015–2019. Drug Trials Snapshots. Summary Report. Five-year summary and analysis of clinical trial participation and demographics. U.S. Food and Drug Administration. https://www.fda.gov/media/143592/download?attachment. Accessed January 8, 2024.

314. https://www.census.gov/quickfacts/fact/table/US/POP010220#POP010220. Accessed January 8, 2024.

315. Myers TL, Augustine EF, Baloga E, Daeschler M, Cannon P, Rowbotham H, Chanoff E; 23andMe Research Team; Jensen-Roberts S, Soto J, Holloway RG, Marras C, Tanner CM, Dorsey ER, Schneider RB. Recruitment for Remote Decentralized Studies in Parkinson's Disease. *J Parkinsons Dis*. 2022;12(1):371–380. doi: 10.3233/JPD-212935. PMID: 34744053; PMCID: PMC8842745.

316. Jones WS, Mulder H, Wruck LM, Pencina MJ, Kripalani S, Muñoz D, Crenshaw DL, Effron MB, Re RN, Gupta K, Anderson RD, Pepine CJ, Handberg EM, Manning BR, Jain SK, Girotra S, Riley D, DeWalt DA, Whittle J, Goldberg YH, Roger VL, Hess R, Benziger CP, Farrehi P, Zhou L, Ford DE, Haynes K, VanWormer JJ, Knowlton KU, Kraschnewski JL, Polonsky TS, Fintel DJ, Ahmad FS, McClay JC, Campbell JR, Bell DS, Fonarow GC, Bradley SM, Paranjape A, Roe MT, Robertson HR, Curtis LH, Sharlow AG, Berdan LG, Hammill BG, Harris DF, Qualls LG, Marquis-Gravel G, Modrow MF, Marcus GM, Carton TW, Nauman E, Waitman LR, Kho AN, Shenkman EA, McTigue KM, Kaushal R, Masoudi FA, Antman EM, Davidson DR, Edgley K, Merritt JG, Brown LS, Zemon DN, McCormick TE 3rd, Alikhaani JD, Gregoire KC, Rothman RL, Harrington RA, Hernandez AF; ADAPTABLE Team. Comparative effectiveness of aspirin dosing in cardiovascular disease. *N Engl J Med*. 2021 May 27;384(21):1981–1990. doi: 10.1056/NEJMoa2102137. Epub 2021 May 15. PMID: 33999548; PMCID: PMC9908069.

317. Sathian B, Asim M, Banerjee I, Pizarro AB, Roy B, van Teijlingen ER, do Nascimento IJB, Alhamad HK. Impact of COVID-19 on clinical trials and clinical research: a systematic review. *Nepal J Epidemiol*. 2020 Sep 30;10(3):878–887. doi: 10.3126/nje.v10i3.31622. PMID: 33042591; PMCID: PMC7538012.

318. Sarraju A, Seninger C, Parameswaran V, Petlura C, Bazouzi T, Josan K, Grewal U, Viethen T, Mundl H, Luithle J, Basobas L, Touros A, Senior MJT, De Lombaert K, Mahaffey KW, Turakhia MP, Dash R. Pandemic-proof recruitment and engagement in a fully decentralized trial in atrial fibrillation patients (DeTAP). *NPJ Digit Med*. 2022 Jun 28;5(1):80. doi: 10.1038/s41746-022-00622-9. PMID: 35764796; PMCID: PMC9240050.

319. Sommer C, Zuccolin D, Arnera V, Schmitz N, Adolfsson P, Colombo N, Gilg R, McDowell B. Building clinical trials around patients: evaluation and comparison of decentralized and conventional site models in patients with low back pain. *Contemp Clin Trials Commun*. 2018 Jun 28;11:120–126. doi: 10.1016/j.conctc.2018.06.008. PMID: 30094387; PMCID: PMC6072894.

320. Dal-Ré R. Unperceived similarities between clinical trials and quantum physics. *Br J Clin Pharmacol*. 2020 Feb;86(2):192–193. doi: 10.1111/bcp.14126. Epub 2020 Jan 14. PMID: 31943305; PMCID: PMC7015734.

321. https://www.fda.gov/media/167696/download. Accessed December 21, 2023.

322. Darmawan I, Bakker C, Brockman TA, Patten CA, Eder M. The role of social media in enhancing clinical trial recruitment: scoping review. *J Med Internet Res*. 2020 Oct 26;22(10):e22810. doi: 10.2196/22810. PMID: 33104015; PMCID: PMC7652693.

323. Møllgård K, Beinlich FRM, Kusk P, Miyakoshi LM, Delle C, Plá V, Hauglund NL, Esmail T, Rasmussen MK, Gomolka RS, Mori Y, Nedergaard M. A mesothelium divides the subarachnoid space into functional compartments. *Science*. 2023 Jan 6;379(6627):84–88. doi: 10.1126/science.adc8810. Epub 2023 Jan 5. PMID: 36603070.

324. Hussain G, Akram R, Anwar H, Sajid F, Iman T, Han HS, Raza C, De Aguilar JG. Adult neurogenesis: a real hope or a delusion? *Neural Regen Res*. 2024 Jan;19(1):6–15. doi: 10.4103/1673-5374.375317. PMID: 37488837.

325. Hore PJ, Mouritsen H. How migrating birds use quantum effects to navigate. *Scientific American.* April 1, 2022.

326. Al-Khalili J, McFadden J. *Life on the Edge: The Coming of Age of Quantum Biology.* Bantam Press;2014.

327. Al-Khalili J, McFadden J. *Life on the Edge: The Coming of Age of Quantum Biology.* Bantam Press;2014.

328. English LK, Ard JD, Bailey RL, Bates M, Bazzano LA, Boushey CJ, Brown C, Butera G, Callahan EH, de Jesus J, Mattes RD, Mayer-Davis EJ, Novotny R, Obbagy JE, Rahavi EB, Sabate J, Snetselaar LG, Stoody EE, Van Horn LV, Venkatramanan S, Heymsfield SB. Evaluation of dietary patterns and all-cause mortality: a systematic review. *JAMA Netw Open.* 2021 Aug 2;4(8):e2122277. doi: 10.1001/jamanetworkopen.2021.22277. PMID: 34463743; PMCID: PMC8408672.

329. https://www.inotivco.com/atherogenic-custom-diets#:~:text=Within%20the%20atherogenic%20literature%2C%20a,and%20 34%25%20sucrose%20by%20weight. Accessed August 10, 2023.

330. Kim Y, Je Y, Giovannucci EL. Association between dietary fat intake and mortality from all-causes, cardiovascular disease, and cancer: a systematic review and meta-analysis of prospective cohort studies. *Clin Nutr.* 2021 Mar;40(3):1060–1070. doi: 10.1016/j. clnu.2020.07.007. Epub 2020 Jul 14. PMID: 32723506.

331. Huang C, Liang Z, Ma J, Hu D, Yao F, Qin P. Total sugar, added sugar, fructose, and sucrose intake and all-cause, cardiovascular, and cancer mortality: a systematic review and dose-response meta-analysis of prospective cohort studies. *Nutrition.* 2023 Jul;111:112032. doi: 10.1016/j.nut.2023.112032. Epub 2023 Mar 16. PMID: 37182401.

332. Visioli F, Mucignat-Caretta C, Anile F, Panaite SA. Traditional and medical applications of fasting. *Nutrients*. 2022 Jan 19;14(3):433. doi: 10.3390/nu14030433. PMID: 35276792; PMCID: PMC8838777.

333. Longo VD, Mattson MP. Fasting: molecular mechanisms and clinical applications. *Cell Metab*. 2014 Feb 4;19(2):181–192. doi: 10.1016/j.cmet.2013.12.008. Epub 2014 Jan 16. PMID: 24440038; PMCID: PMC3946160.

334. de Cabo R, Mattson MP. Effects of Intermittent Fasting on Health, Aging, and Disease. *N Engl J Med*. 2019 Dec 26;381(26):2541–2551. doi: 10.1056/NEJMra1905136. Erratum in: *N Engl J Med*. 2020 Jan 16;382(3):298. Erratum in: *N Engl J Med*. 2020 Mar 5;382(10):978. PMID: 31881139.

335. Goldhamer A, Lisle D, Parpia B, Anderson SV, Campbell TC. Medically supervised water-only fasting in the treatment of hypertension. *J Manipulative Physiol Ther*. 2001 Jun;24(5):335–339. doi: 10.1067/mmt.2001.115263. PMID: 11416824.

336. Ko Y. Sebastian Kneipp and the natural cure movement of Germany: between naturalism and modern medicine. *Korean Journal of Medical History*. 2016 Dec 31;25(3):557–590.

337. Brenner IK, Castellani JW, Gabaree C, Young AJ, Zamecnik J, Shephard RJ, Shek PN. Immune changes in humans during cold exposure: effects of prior heating and exercise. *J Appl Physiol* (1985). 1999 Aug;87(2):699–710. doi: 10.1152/jappl.1999.87.2.699. PMID: 10444630.

338. Stick C, Rischewski C, Eggert P, Scheewe S. Änderungen der Nasenschleimhautdurchblutung bei infektanfälligen Kindern nach einer Klimakur an der See. Physikalische Medizin, Rehabilitationsmedizin, Kurortmedizin. 2000 Feb;10(01):6–10.

339. House Hearing, 110 Congress. U.S. Government Publishing Office. The adequacy of FDA to assure the safety of the National Drug Supply. Feb 13, Mar 22, 2007. See https://www.govinfo.gov/content/pkg/CHRG-110hhrg35502/html/CHRG-110hhrg35502.htm. Accessed May 15, 2023. See also compelling testimony from Dr. Steven Nissen in this hearing.

340. Parasrampuria S, Beleche T. FDA User Fees: examining changes in medical product development and economic benefits. Washington, DC: Office of the Assistant Secretary for Planning and Evaluation, U.S. Department of Health and Human Services. March 2023.

341. Frank C, Himmelstein DU, Woolhandler S, Bor DH, Wolfe SM, Heymann O, Zallman L, Lasser KE. Era of faster FDA drug approval has also seen increased black-box warnings and market withdrawals. *Health Aff* (Millwood). 2014;33(8):1453–1459.

342. Black Currant oil decision: appeal to U.S. Supreme Court. April 19, 1993. The Tan Sheet. See: https://pink.pharmaintelligence.informa.com/PS081338/BLACK-CURRANT-OIL-DECISION-APPEAL-TO-US-SUPREME-COURT. Accessed May 15, 2023.

343. F.D.A. steps up effort to control vitamin claims. August 9, 1992. *New York Times*. https://www.nytimes.com/1992/08/09/us/fda-steps-up-effort-to-control-vitamin-claims.html. Accessed May 15, 2023.

344. https://www.wholefoodsmagazine.com/articles/3732-industry-trailblazers-and-the-fight-for-health-freedom. Accessed May 23, 2023.

345. https://www.congress.gov/bill/103rd-congress/senate-bill/784. Accessed March 22, 2024.

346. https://www.fda.gov/drugs/news-events-human-drugs/fdas-regulation-dietary-supplements-dr-cara-welch#:~:text=The%20dietary%20supplement%20market%20is,the%20public%20about%20dietary%20supplements. Accessed March 25, 2024.

347. https://www.fda.gov/about-fda/center-drug-evaluation-and-research-cder/what-botanical-drug. Accessed July 18, 2023.

348. https://www.ftc.gov/system/files/ftc_gov/pdf/rks_substantiation_pno_statement_lk_ab_final.pdf. Accessed March 8, 2024.

349. https://www.ftc.gov/news-events/news/press-releases/2023/04/ftc-warns-almost-700-marketing-companies-they-could-face-civil-penalties-if-they-cant-back-their. Accessed March 22, 2024.

350. https://www.ftc.gov/business-guidance/resources/health-products-compliance-guidance. Accessed March 22, 2024.

351. Hanin L. Why statistical inference from clinical trials is likely to generate false and irreproducible results. *BMC Med Res Methodol.* 2017 Aug 22;17(1):127. doi: 10.1186/s12874-017-0399-0. PMID: 28830371; PMCID: PMC5568363.

352. Ioannidis JP. Contradicted and initially stronger effects in highly cited clinical research. *JAMA.* 2005 Jul 13;294(2):218–228. doi: 10.1001/jama.294.2.218. PMID: 16014596.

353. htttps://www.congress.gov/bill/103rd-congress/senate-bill/784. Accessed March 22, 2024.

354. htttps://www.congress.gov/bill/103rd-congress/senate-bill/784. Accessed March 22, 2024.